FLUIDS and ELECTROLYTES

EDITION 2

FLUIDS and ELECTROLYTES:

A PRACTICAL APPROACH

VIOLET R. STROOT, R.N.

Assistant Instructor and Preceptorship Coordinator, Nurse Clinician Department, College of Health Related Professions, Wichita State University, Wichita, Kansas. Guest Lecturer in Fluids and Electrolytes. Formerly Project Nurse, Fluid, Electrolyte and Renal Program, Kansas Regional Medical Program, St. Francis Hospital, Wichita, Kansas.

CARLA A. LEE, R.N., B.S.N., M.A., Ed.S.

Assistant Professor, Chairperson Project Director, Nurse Clinician Department, College of Health Related Professions, Wichita State University, Wichita, Kansas. Formerly Educational Assistant, Wesley Medical Center School of Nursing; Nurse Lecturer, Fluid, Electrolyte and Renal Program, Kansas Regional Medical Program, St. Francis Hospital, Wichita, Kansas.

C. ANN SCHAPER, B.A.

Media Consultant, Project Success, Butler County Community Junior College, El Dorado, Kansas. Formerly Writer, Audio Visual Systems, Wesley Medical Center, Wichita, Kansas.

F. A. DAVIS COMPANY, Philadelphia

Library of Congress Cataloging in Publication Data
Stroot, Violet R.

   Fluids and electrolytes.

   Bibliography: p.
   Includes index.
   1. Body fluid disorders. 2. Water-electrolyte
imbalances. 3. Body fluids. 4. Water-electrolyte
balance (Physiology). I. Lee, Carla A., joint author.
II. Schaper, C. Ann, joint author. III. Title.
[DNLM: 1. Water-electrolyte balance — Nursing texts.
2. Water-electrolyte imbalance — Nursing texts. WD220
S924]
RC630.S77 1977   612'.01522   76-53014
ISBN 0-8036-8206-9

Dedicated to

THOMAS J. LUELLEN, M.D.

Preface

There is no greater delight to an author than to gather the comments and critiques of his reading audience and set forth upon a revision of the original work. Revision has the dual purpose of meeting the professional needs of the reading constituency and providing new and updated material.

In this edition we increased the size of the book, thereby allowing room for personal notes in the margins. Note pages have also been supplied at the ends of chapters. The material from the first edition was evaluated for currency and clarity and the bibliography was expanded.

Most important, there are two new chapters. A chapter on Burns has been added to the Clinical Situation section. Much of burn therapy is dependent on an in-depth understanding of fluid and electrolyte balance. A chapter on Intravenous Therapy has been added to the Nursing Techniques section. This subject is relevant since it is both a system for altering the fluid level in the body and a technique for the administration of chemicals directly to the circulatory system.

The first edition evolved from a federally funded (Kansas Regional Medical Program) teaching project in Fluid, Electrolyte, and Renal Problems and from the need expressed by these students for a simplified book using the same style and encompassing the same material as our seminar presentations. With this approach the participants found it easier to assimilate the material and to relate it directly to everyday health care problems.

The philosophy of this second edition remains the same and can be summed up in two words: "pragmatic" and "simplified." It is not designed as a comprehensive work but rather as a book that the health team member can relate directly to the clinical situation. The text lays the groundwork in fluid and electrolyte balances. Should the reader then desire a more thorough background in theory, he can refer to the numerous, more comprehensive and complex texts that already exist.

The major objectives of this book are to identify principles related to fluids and electrolytes within the human body and to apply these principles to the clinical situation. The desired result is that nurses will use this text to plan for and provide quality nursing care. In addition, the text will serve as a guideline for evaluating current health care practices.

Although this text is especially directed to the nurse as a continuing student and nursing practitioner, we also envision the use of the text by other members of the health team, i.e., licensed practical nurses, medical technologists, nutritionists, physicians, physician assistants, and therapists.

Chapter 1 provides the foundation for the rest of the book. The remaining chapters are organized to include information about causative factors, recognition of signs and symptoms or impending problems, laboratory tests, treatment, and nurse's responsibilities. Throughout the chapters, we include illustrations for clarification and case studies to encourage application of new knowledge to clinical situations.

Quizzes are provided to assist the reader in evaluating his knowledge. Case study and quiz answers are included in the appendices so the reader can validate his answers. A glossary is provided to assist the reader in acquiring a working knowledge of terminology. The words listed in the glossary are in boldface type the first time they appear in the text. The appendices contain supplementary but valuable material.

We dedicate this book to Thomas J. Luellen, M.D., who continually expressed his belief that nurses need to learn and apply this information in the clinical setting.

Without the tremendous support and patience of our families, this book would not have become a reality. To Leo, Ted, Mike, Steve, Connie, and Ricky Stroot, to Gordon Larry Lee, and to James, Kelli, and Scott Schaper, we owe a special thank you.

Violet R. Stroot
Carla A. Lee
C. Ann Schaper

Contents

*Chapter is supplemented with Case Studies.

x   Contents

Section VI: Nursing Techniques

Appendices

SECTION I

INTRODUCTION

1

The Basics

Approximately 60 per cent of the total weight of the human body is composed of fluid. Respiration, metabolism, digestion, excretion, and life itself are affected by the solutes or **electrolytes*** contained in this fluid. An imbalance of these electrolytes or fluid can seriously jeopardize a patient's life.

An astute nurse can help the patient maintain or regain normal balance. In nearly every case of possible fluid or electrolyte imbalance, the nurse can prevent a patient's condition from deteriorating by utilizing all the steps of the nursing process. This includes the observation of clinical manifestations of fluid and electrolyte imbalances, assessment of the patients needs (both actual and potential), planning and implementation of appropriate nursing actions, and evaluation of the effectiveness of all the above aspects of the treatment. Therefore the nurse must possess enough knowledge of body fluid disturbances to make an intelligent nursing diagnosis and care plan.

The primary emphases of this book are on *recognizing* the signs and symptoms of fluid and electrolyte imbalance as they appear in the clinical situation and on *taking the necessary steps* to decrease the incidence of **morbidity** and **mortality** among patients who develop these problems. In other words, this book will deal more with practical application than with theory. However, some background in the physiology of fluid and electrolyte function is necessary. The next few pages provide this background and the basic terminology needed to better comprehend the following chapters.

Body Fluids

Fluid in the body is primarily water (H_2O). Important **solutes,** without which the body could not maintain **homeostasis,** are dissolved in this water (called the **solution** or **solvent**). Solutes found in the body's fluid vary according to the area they occupy. There are two basic fluid compartments: **intracellular** and **extracellular**. The intracellular compartment is the area within the cell and is primarily water. The extracellular compartment is composed of the **interstitial** area, which is the area around the cells, and the **intravascular** area, which is the area within the blood vessels. **Extracellular fluid** is primarily saline (Na^+, Cl^-, and H_2O).

*Words listed in the Glossary are in boldface type the first time they appear in the text.

**Fluid and
Electrolyte
Transportation**

There are two types of transport systems: passive and active.

Passive Transport Systems

Body fluid movement takes place by means of three *passive* transport systems: **diffusion, filtration,** and **osmosis.** Diffusion is based on the principle that **molecules** and **ions** flow from an area of higher concentration of solute to an area of lower concentration in order to establish an equilibrium (Fig. 1-1). Diffusion is a passive transport system motivated by the concentration of the solute.

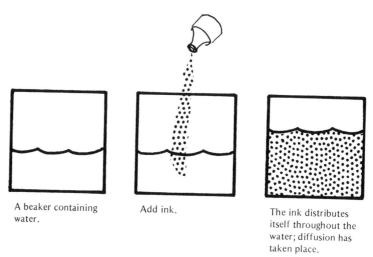

A beaker containing water.

Add ink.

The ink distributes itself throughout the water; diffusion has taken place.

Figure 1-1.   Diffusion.

Filtration is the movement of solute and solvent by **hydrostatic pressure.** Hydrostatic pressure is the force exerted by the weight of a solution. The movement is from an area of greater pressure to an area of lesser pressure (Fig. 1-2).

Osmosis is the diffusion of a solution or solvent through a **semipermeable membrane** and is the process by which fluids move to and from intracellular and extracellular areas. In the human body, free water molecules move by osmosis (Fig. 1-3). The combined actions of hydrostatic pressure, which moves water and minute solutes, and **osmolarity,** which moves water, provide the transportation system for the interaction of the body's fluids and electrolytes. The term osmolarity refers to the concentration of a solute in a solvent.

The concentration of solutes dissolved in the body fluid affects the movement of the fluid. This effect, called **osmotic pressure,** causes fluid to move in both directions simultaneously. The variation in concentration of solution causes greater movement in one direction but does not preclude movement in the other direction. The osmotic pressures of electrolytes in a solution differ. There are two basic divisions of osmotic pressure: **crystalloid,** relating to dissolved ions which can pass through a membrane, and **colloid,** relating to gelatinous substances which in healthy conditions do not pass through a

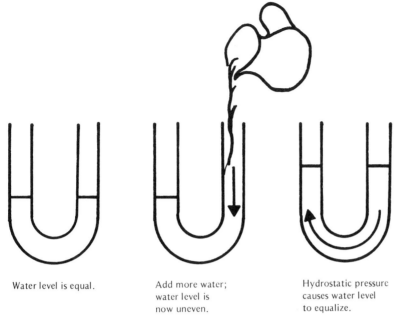

Water level is equal.

Add more water;
water level is
now uneven.

Hydrostatic pressure
causes water level
to equalize.

Figure 1-2.   Hydrostatic pressure.

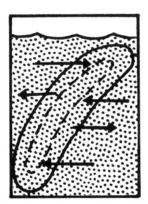

Figure 1-3.   Osmosis. A hot dog placed in water demonstrates osmosis. The hot dog will expand as water molecules pass through the semipermeable skin. Once an equilibrium has been established the molecules will move freely in and out.

membrane. The solution itself may be either **hypertonic, hypotonic,** or **isotonic.** A hypertonic solution exerts *greater* osmotic pressure than the solution to which it is compared. A hypotonic solution exerts *less* osmotic pressure than the solution to which it is compared. In an isotonic solution, the osmotic pressure exerted is *equal* to the solution to which it is compared (Fig. 1-4). In the human body blood **plasma** is the isotonic standard (0.9 per cent). For example, red blood cells placed in a beaker of normal **saline** solution are isotonic. The osmotic pressures on both sides of the cell membrane are equal (Fig. 1-4B). These same red blood cells placed in a beaker with a highly saline solution would release free water molecules. This free water passes through the semipermeable membrane from the cell into the saline solution, causing the cells to shrink, **crenation.** The highly saline solution is a hypertonic solution (Fig. 1-4A). If the red blood cells are

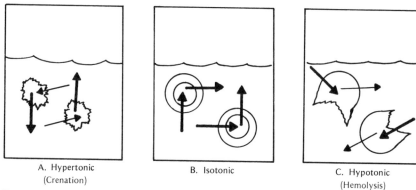

| A. Hypertonic | B. Isotonic | C. Hypotonic |
| (Crenation) | | (Hemolysis) |

Figure 1-4. Comparison of solution (large arrows indicate greater movement). (A) Osmotic pressure or pull of the solution surrounding cell causes more water to move out of the cell than into the cell. (B) Solution and cells have equal movement of fluid. (C) Osmotic pressure or pull of the solution within the cell causes more water to move into the cell than out of the cell.

placed in a beaker of pure or distilled water, the free water molecules would pass through the semipermeable membrane from the water into the cell causing the cells to expand and eventually rupture, **hemolysis.** The distilled water is a hypotonic solution (Fig. 1-4C).

Active Transport System

The principle of the *active* transport system is that substances can be moved from an area of lower concentration of solute to an area of higher concentration with the expenditure of energy. Scientists have only theoretically established how this process takes place.

Electrolytes

Electrolytes are the chemical compounds dissolved in the body fluids. They are called electrolytes because they contain small electrically charged particles called ions. Pure, distilled water has no electrolytes and does not conduct an electric current. If a small amount of sodium chloride is added to the distilled water, the resulting salt solution does conduct electricity. When dissolved in water, many acids, bases, and salts **ionize** and become electrolytes.

When electrolytes are dissolved in water, they split into electrically charged atoms or groups of atoms. It is these atoms and groups of atoms that are referred to by the term ion. Since ions have an electrical charge, they are classified as either negative or positive. Negative ions are called **anions;** positive ions are called **cations.**

Table 1-1 lists the primary electrolytes found in the human body and their chemical symbol and function.

Electrolytes are important constituents of body fluids that serve vital functions. The health team needs to know the quantity of various electrolytes in body fluids as well as the patient's intake and output of electrolytes.

There are several ways to express electrolyte quantities. The term **milliequivalent** has come into widespread use because it is convenient and precise and because all electrolyte quantities can be expressed on the basis of their combining activity. The system of milliequivalents makes it possible to compare one compound directly with another. Electrolytes are usually measured in milliequivalents per liter (mEq/L).

TABLE 1-1. ELECTROLYTES, CHEMICAL SYMBOLS, AND FUNCTIONS

Electrolyte	Chemical Symbol	Function
Cations		
Sodium	Na^+	Major extracellular cation; fluid balance; crystalloid osmotic pressure
Potassium	K^+	Major intracellular cation; neuromuscular excitability; acid-base balance
Calcium	Ca^{++}	Neuromuscular irritability; blood clotting; bone structure
Magnesium	Mg^{++}	Enzyme systems
Anions		
Chloride	Cl^-	Major extracellular anion; fluid balance; crystalloid osmotic pressure
Bicarbonate	HCO_3^-	Acid-base balance
Proteinates		Colloid osmotic pressure; acid-base balance
Organic acids		Intermediary cellular metabolism
Phosphates	HPO_4^{--}	Major intracellular anion
Sulfate	SO_4^{--}	Protein metabolism

Acid-Base

The hydrogen ion exists in very small quantities in the human body, yet it has the crucial task of maintaining the acid-base balance at the normal 20:1 ratio of bicarbonate to carbonic acid. Acid-base refers to the acidity or alkalinity of body fluid and is represented by the term **pH.** An *excess* of hydrogen ions results in **acidosis.** A *deficit* of hydrogen ions results in **alkalosis.**

The normal pH (hydrogen concentration) of the extracellular fluid is between 7.35 and 7.45. A pH above 7.45 indicates alkalosis; a pH below 7.35 indicates acidosis. When the level is over 7.8 or below 7.0, death usually occurs. Acidosis and alkalosis can result from either metabolic or respiratory malfunctions.

Nursing Challenges

All the terms and concepts presented in this introduction will be explained in greater depth in the chapters that follow. Concepts such as diffusion, osmotic pressure, electrolytes, and milliequivalents are directly related to the clinical situation and the problems the nurse meets in day-to-day nursing care.

A great deal of emphasis will be placed on recognition of signs and symptoms because usually they are the first indications of a fluid or electrolyte imbalance. Some of the signs and symptoms will be common to other ailments, but many times the signs or symptoms the nurse normally associates with another ailment can also indicate a fluid or electrolyte imbalance, as for example, a symptom as common as weakness. In many cases imbalance can be caused by other diseases and sometimes even by the treatment itself. Therefore the nurse should always consider the possibility of fluid and electrolyte imbalance when treating a patient.

The nurse's observations and actions should begin with the patient's admission to the hospital, for it is at this time that a baseline is established from the patient's weight, blood pressure, temperature, pulse, and respiration. The nurse should observe the patient and record such data as **edema, sensorium, skin turgor,** weakness, and other clinical signs both upon admission and during hospitalization. As the nurse becomes skillful in recognizing and anticipating circumstances that can develop into serious situations, "nursing problems" will become "nursing challenges."

BIBLIOGRAPHY

Abbott Laboratories: Fluid and Electrolytes, Some Practical Guides to Clinical Use. Abbott Laboratories, North Chicago, 1969.

Baxter Laboratories: The Fundamentals of Body Water and Electrolytes. Travenol Laboratories, Inc., Morton Grove, Illinois, 1967.

Bordicks, K. J.: Patterns of Shock. The Macmillan Company, New York, 1965.

Condon, R. E., and Nyhus, L. M.: Manual of Surgical Therapeutics, ed. 3. Little, Brown and Company, Boston, 1975.

Goldberger, E.: A Primer of Water, Electrolyte, and Acid-Base Syndrome, ed. 5. Lea and Febiger, Philadelphia, 1975.

Guyton, A. C.: Function of the Human Body, ed. 4. W. B. Saunders Company, Philadelphia, 1974.

Kee, J. L.: Fluids and Electrolytes with Clinical Applications: A Programmed Approach. John Wiley and Sons, Inc., New York, 1971.

Mason, E. E.: Fluid, Electrolyte, and Nutrient Therapy in Surgery. Lea and Febiger, Philadelphia, 1974.

Metheny, N. M., and Snively, W. D., Jr.: Nurses' Handbook of Fluid Balance, ed. 2. J. B. Lippincott Company, Philadelphia, 1974.

Scribner, B. H., and Burnell, J. M.: The Teaching Syllabus for the Course on Fluid and Electrolyte Balance, ed. 7. University of Washington, Seattle, 1969.

Snipes, R.: Statistical Mechanical Theory of the Electrolytic Transport of Non-electrolytes. Springer-Verlag Inc., New York, 1973.

Taber's Cyclopedic Medical Dictionary, ed. 13. F. A. Davis Company, Philadelphia, 1977.

NOTES

NOTES

SECTION II

FLUIDS

2

Extracellular Fluid: Excess and Deficit

Body fluids are distributed proportionately between two fluid compartments: the extracellular and the intracellular (see Ch. 3). Extracellular fluid is sometimes called saline and intracellular fluid is called water. The primary electrolytes and the major regulators of fluid and electrolyte balance in the extracellular compartment are **sodium** and **chloride.**

Fluid Distribution

The fluids in the extracellular compartment represent about 20 percent of the total body weight. A 165-pound (75 **kilogram*, 75 kg**) man will have about 15 liters (L) of extracellular fluid in his body. This is approximately one third of the total body fluid. These 15 liters of extracellular fluid are divided between the interstitial and the intravascular areas. The interstitial area contains approximately 12 liters of fluid, whereas the intravascular fluid or plasma contains approximately 3 liters. An additional 2.5 liters of cellular material are not part of the saline fluid. The major difference between interstitial and intravascular fluids is that intravascular fluid contains more protein or colloids.

Electrolyte Distribution

The major electrolytes of the extracellular fluid **(ECF)** compartment are the cation sodium and the anions chloride, **bicarbonate,** and **proteinate.** The total number of ions found in the extracellular fluid is 308 mEq/L. Their distribution is shown in Figure 2-1, representing primarily the plasma distribution.

Fluid and Electrolyte Losses

All living persons have daily obligatory losses of approximately 2500 cubic centimeters (2.5 liters), termed sensible and insensible. **Sensible losses** are those of which an individual is aware, such as urination. **Insensible losses,** such as imperceptible perspiration, occur without the individual's awareness. The immediate sensible-insensible losses are from the extracellular fluid compartment.

Sensible Losses. Urination accounts for the loss of approximately 1500 cubic centimeters (cc) of extracellular fluid during each 24-hour period.

---

*See Conversion Chart in Appendix.

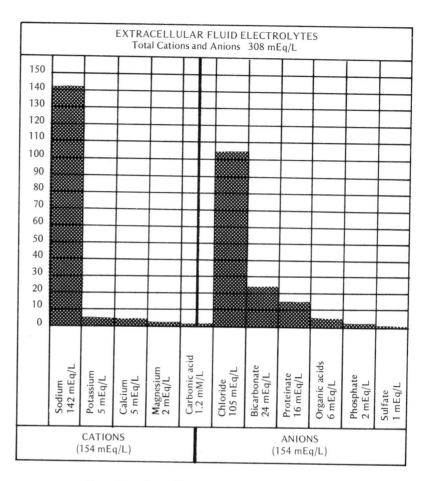

Figure 2-1. Extracellular fluid electrolyte distribution.

Urinary excretions are extracted from the extracellular fluid, but the electrolyte losses are selective. Under normal circumstances the kidneys discard only excess electrolytes. Approximately 50 mEq of sodium, 40 mEq of potassium, and 90 mEq of chloride are lost in each liter (1000 cc) of urine and must be replaced.

Insensible Losses. Approximately 1000 cc of extracellular fluid are lost every 24 hours through the skin and lungs. There are no electrolytes in the fluid lost by imperceptible perspiration. However, depending on climatic changes and increased activity, fluid losses can increase to the point of causing an electrolyte loss. These losses can reach serious levels if perspiration is profuse, as in **febrile** conditions. As much as one liter of fluid with electrolytes can be lost with each episode of profuse **diaphoresis.** Insensible losses occur without regard to intake or losses through other processes.

Not all secretions are lost from the body. Digestive juices are secreted and reabsorbed at the rate of approximately 8000 cc every 24 hours. This gastrointestinal fluid contains sodium and chloride (50 to 100 mEq/L) and potassium (5 to 10mEq/L). All food and fluid ingested into the body, excluding undigestible waste by-products, are absorbed into the extracellular fluid. During normal body function, gastrointestinal fluids are reabsorbed. It is important to note, however, that during illness they are often lost from the body, causing fluid and electrolyte imbalances.

EXTRACELLU-LAR FLUID EXCESS

An electrolyte report will not indicate whether or not a patient has an extracellular fluid excess or deficit. **Serum** electrolyte values can be normal, high, or low in the presence of either an excess or deficit of extracellular fluid (Fig. 2-2). Thus imbalances must be detected through the clinical condition and history of the patient.

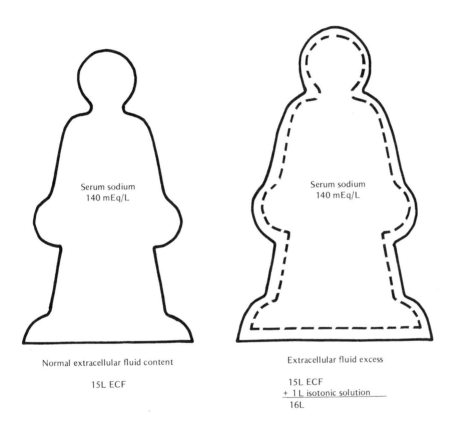

Serum sodium
140 mEq/L

Serum sodium
140 mEq/L

Normal extracellular fluid content

15L ECF

Extracellular fluid excess

15L ECF
+ 1 L isotonic solution
16L

Figure 2-2. Expanded extracellular compartment. Note that the extracellular compartment has expanded to 16 liters but the serum sodium reading remains the same.

Causes of Extracellular Fluid Excess

In extracellular fluid excess the compartment becomes expanded. Extracellular fluid excess most commonly occurs when the kidneys are not functioning properly. This dysfunction may be caused by primary renal disease or by conditions that result in decreased renal blood flow, such as cardiac insufficiency or liver disease.

Table 2-1 lists additional causes of altered functions leading to extracellular fluid excess.

TABLE 2-1. CAUSES OF EXTRACELLULAR FLUID EXCESS

Cause	Altered Function
Cardiac insufficiency	Decreased renal perfusion due to inadequate cardiac pump; thus fluid retained by the body
Cirrhosis; ascites	Decreased hepatic perfusion; decreased renal blood flow
Protein depletion	Insufficient intravascular protein resulting in movement of fluid into interstitial area
Rapid administration of intravenous saline	Pulmonary edema and congestive heart failure
Stress; steroid therapy	Release or administration of **aldosterone,** causing sodium reabsorption by the kidney tubules
Renal disease	Decreased renal perfusion

Recognition

Merely knowing what causes extracellular fluid excess is not enough. It is necessary for the nurse to be able to recognize the signs and symptoms that indicate the existence of extracellular fluid excess.

There are several signs that should alert the nurse to possible extracellular fluid excess. True **pitting edema** always indicates extracellular fluid excess. Edema is an expansion of the **interstitial fluid** space. The body can transport this fluid back into the intravascular space by improved circulation or drugs. These excess fluids are then excreted via the kidneys. Other signs are excessive weight gain (a weight gain of 2.2 pounds equals one liter of fluid retention); elevated blood pressure (which may also be caused by other problems); and **dyspnea,** which, however, is not always present with the condition of excess extracellular fluid. Neck vein distention may also be noted. Central venous pressure is normal or elevated because of increased intravascular volume.

Laboratory Tests

Although there is no electrolyte test to show extracellular fluid excess, laboratory tests can have diagnostic value. The **hematocrit (HCT)** may be normal or low. Since hematocrit is measured in percent of red blood cells per volume of fluid, it will usually read low in an extracellular fluid excess because the amount of red blood cells remains unchanged in an increased volume of extracellular fluid. Urine sodium may be low due to sodium retention. Serum sodium may be high, low or normal; this test does *not* indicate either an excess or deficit of extracellular fluid.

Treatment

The treatment for extracellular fluid excess consists of the administration of **diuretics,** restriction of sodium and fluid intake, and treatment of the underlying cause.

The nurse's observations can be very important to the physician in assessing the fluid status of the patient and planning replacement fluids. An accurate intake-output record is essential. (See the sample Intake and Output Record in Appendix 3.) Take accurate body weights, preferably with a balance scale. Weigh the patient under the same conditions each day. Signs of edema must be observed and reported. Elderly patients may develop **dependent edema** with relatively little excess fluid. In patients in a constant supine position, edema can first be recognized in the sacral area. A patient in a supine position can have an increase of 4 to 8 liters of fluid without detectable edema. Avoid overly rapid infusion of intravenous fluids to prevent extracellular fluid excess (see Chapter 23). Patients maintained exclusively on intravenous fluids should lose about one-half pound (0.23 kg) daily. Observe the patient for signs of dyspnea. Check the patient's blood pressure daily or more frequently for comparison. Blood pressure usually increases as extracellular fluid excess increases. Conversely, blood pressure will decrease as the extracellular fluid level returns to normal. Report all signs and symptoms of extracellular fluid excess to the physician.

When diuretics are used, observe the patient for evidence of potassium depletion, elevated blood urea nitrogen (BUN), metabolic alkalosis, and extracellular fluid depletion. Potassium can be replaced by diet or intravenous therapy. Restrict sodium and fluid intake as directed by the physician. Observe neck veins for distention. Be aware of conditions such as those listed in Table 2-1 which predispose the patient to extracellular fluid excess. (A patient with normal heart and kidneys can tolerate an extracellular fluid excess quite well, whereas a patient with poorly functioning heart or kidneys cannot.)

In summary, the nurse's responsibilities are as follows:

Maintain accurate intake and output record.
Obtain accurate body weight measurements.
Observe for pulmonary and pitting edema.
Regulate intravenous fluid as directed or maintain "keep-open" rate.
Restrict sodium/water intake as ordered.
Observe for potassium depletion and replace as needed.
Monitor vital signs.

In extracellular fluid deficit, the extracellular compartment becomes contracted (Fig. 2-3). Extracellular fluid deficit occurs when fluid is lost from the body or when it collects in a **"third space."** A third space is any area where extracellular fluid accumulates and becomes physiologically unavailable to the body. In other words, the fluid cannot be drawn back into circulation as extracellular fluid because body mechanics cannot transport it from the place where it has accumulated. It is often removed by use of tubes. For example, **ascites** is a third space fluid accumulation.

Extracellular fluid deficit is most commonly caused by fluids lost through the gastrointestinal tract. Additional possible causes are listed in Table 2-2. Normally the fluids in the gastrointestinal tract are reabsorbed, but under certain circumstances these fluids are lost from the body, such as in vomiting and diarrhea.

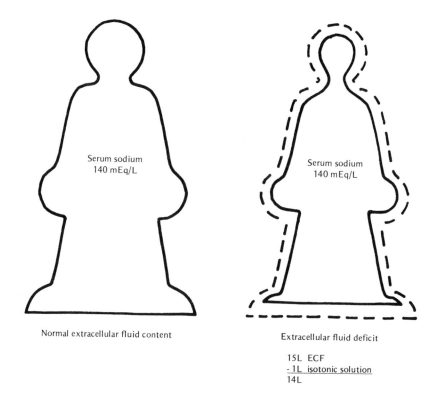

Figure 2-3.   Contracted extracellular compartment. Note that the extracellular compartment has contracted to 14 liters but the serum sodium reading remains the same.

Early recognition of extracellular fluid deficit is vital to the patient's life. After blood loss and **hypoproteinemia,** extracellular fluid deficit is the most common cause of **hypovolemia.** Severe extracellular fluid deficit may impair renal function and may lead to **shock.** (Shock is discussed in detail in Chapter 18.)

Recognition

As with an extracellular fluid excess, there is no electrolyte test that shows that a deficit is developing or has developed. Signs and symptoms exhibited by the patient can provide this information, and other laboratory tests are beneficial.

These signs and symptoms may indicate other physical problems as well, but the alert nurse should consider the possibility of extracellular fluid deficit when any of these signs or symptoms appear. During extracellular fluid deficit, changes in the **postural blood pressure** may occur. When the systolic blood pressure is at least 10 millimeters (mm) lower in a sitting or standing position than in a supine position, this can indicate an extracellular fluid deficit. Poor skin turgor, decreased fullness of the neck veins, nausea, vomiting, weakness, and **anorexia** are all signs or symptoms that indicate a possible extracellular fluid deficit. In severe cases, **oliguria** occurs. Oliguria is a urinary output below 20 cc in 1 hour, 160 cc in 8 hours, or 480 cc in 24 hours.

TABLE 2-2. CAUSES OF EXTRACELLULAR FLUID DEFICIT

Cause	Altered Function
GASTROINTESTINAL	
Vomiting	Reverse **peristalsis** causes loss of extracellular secretions which contain large amounts of sodium and chloride
Diarrhea	Increased forward peristalsis shortens absorption period, preventing ECF absorption
Fistulous drainage	Tubelike passageway between the gastrointestinal (GI) tract and an *external* surface allowing loss of ECF
Gastrointestinal suction	Evacuation of ECF by mechanical means, such as Levin or Cantor tubes
Excessive tap water enemas	Hypotonic solution draws electrolytes from ECF, causing saline loss when expelled
RENAL	
Overzealous use of diuretics	Excessive loss of Na, Cl, and H_2O; salt-losing nephritis
DIAPHORESIS	Saline loss
THIRD SPACE	
Peritonitis	Fluid accumulation in the peritoneal cavity due to an infectious and/or inflammatory process
Intestinal obstruction	Fluid accumulation within intestines due to decreased or absent peristalsis
Postoperative condition	Fluid moves into traumatized operative site due to local inflammatory stress response
Thrombophlebitis	Blood clot(s) with inflammation in a vein with resulting venous obstruction
Acute pancreatitis	Inflammatory response with fluid pulled into the inflamed site
Ascites	Serous fluid accumulation in the peritoneal cavity related to interference with portal circulation
Fistulous drainage	Tubelike passageway between the GI tract and *internal* adjacent cavity allowing loss of ECF
Burns	Fluid accumulation in blisters or interstitial space [Fluid may be lost due to evaporation (white bleeding), which is not a third space accumulation.]

Laboratory Tests

Some laboratory tests can help confirm a diagnosis of extracellular fluid deficit. The hematocrit is usually elevated because the number of red blood cells remains unchanged in a decreased volume of extracellular fluid, i.e., the per cent of red blood cells is elevated. Usually the protein count is also elevated. An elevated protein count, like an elevated hematocrit, is a result of the protein content remaining unchanged in a decreased amount of fluid.

Urinary sodium is decreased. A diagnosis of extracellular fluid deficit can be eliminated if the urinary sodium level is above 50 mEq/L and the kidneys are functioning normally. The serum sodium level can be normal, high, or low, as this is not indicative of either extracellular fluid deficit or excess.

Treatment

There are two basic steps in treating an extracellular fluid deficit: (1) correct the causes contributing to the fluid loss, and (2) replace the fluid.

Nurse's Responsibilities

Maintain accurate intake-output records. All gastrointestinal losses are measured and recorded. Be alert to the amount of urine output. A decreased urine output can indicate that the blood volume is insufficient to perfuse the kidneys. The lack of kidney perfusion may cause oliguira to develop. The nurse should also watch closely for and record the incidence of diaphoresis and the number of linen changes. Each episode of profuse diaphoresis, with subsequent linen/clothing change, may represent the loss of one liter of extracellular fluid.

Accurately recorded body weight is an excellent guide to fluid status. Weight gain that accompanies a third space accumulation should not be mistaken for an *increase* in extracellular fluid, because this fluid cannot be utilized by the body and is therefore considered lost. It is important to accurately measure fluid accumulation areas (limbs, abdomen, etc.). Mark these areas clearly and measure at the same point with the same tape measure each time. An increase of one inch on the upper thigh, for example, can indicate that one half of the total blood volume available to the body has been lost and accumulated in a third space.

The gastric tubes should be irrigated with a **normal saline** solution, and the amount recorded on the intake-output record unless an equal amount is withdrawn immediately after it is instilled. Patients who have gastric suction should receive only limited amounts of ice chips and water. Any ingested ice or water should be carefully measured and recorded.

In summary, the nurse's responsibilities are as follows:

Maintain intake and output record.
Obtain accurate body weight measurements.
Measure "third space" fluid accumulation areas.
Observe for vital sign changes.
Monitor intravenous fluids and oral fluids as ordered.

Be alert to conditions that can lead to extracellular fluid deficit and be aware of the serious results—shock, oliguria, renal failure, death—should a deficit be allowed to continue. The informed, knowledgeable nurse will recognize the signs and symptoms of extracellular fluid deficit as it develops and will provide accurate and complete information to the physician so that therapeutic planning can be initiated.

A 67-year-old man was hospitalized with a diagnosis of congestive heart failure. He exhibited the signs and symptoms recorded by the nurse as follows:

Signs: pitting edema, appeared alert and well-oriented, vital signs normal.

Symptoms: **orthopnea,** shortness of breath, weakness, loss of appetite, and loss of weight in spite of the edema.

Admission orders:

1200 calorie diet, 500 mg sodium diet	EKG
Esidrix tab. i qid po	Mercuhydrin 2 cc IM stat
KCl drams ii qid po	Daily weight
Digoxin 0.125 mg qod	Intake and output
SMA 6, CBC in AM	Pulse and blood pressure tid

1. List the signs and symptoms that suggest a fluid imbalance. With what specific imbalance are these associated?

2. Which fluid/electrolyte imbalances commonly occur in congestive heart failure? What situations cause the development of these imbalances?

3. The laboratory test results were: HCT 31%; BUN 26 mg %; Na 136 mEq/L; CO_2 30 mEq/L; Cl 90.8 mEq/L; K 3.1 mEq/L. List the abnormal laboratory value† and state the cause for each of the abnormalities.

4. Four days later the HCT was 35%, K was 3.6 mEq/L, and weight measurement revealed a four pound loss. Why was the HCT higher at this time?

*For answers to Case Study Questions, see Appendix 4.
†See Appendix 2 for normal laboratory values.

Quiz 2.1*

A 67-year-old man was hospitalized with a diagnosis of congestive heart failure. He appeared alert, well-oriented, and his vital signs were normal. The nurse recorded the presence of pitting edema, and the patient complained of orthopnea, shortness of breath, weakness, loss of appetite, and loss of weight.

Check the one correct response:
1. True pitting edema is always a sign of:
_____ a. Extracellular fluid deficit
_____ b. Potassium excess
_____ c. Extracellular fluid excess
2. Hematrocrit was 31 per cent on admission. Four days later it was 35 per cent, and the patient had lost four pounds. Hematocrit was higher because:
_____ a. Extracellular fluid increased
_____ b. Extracellular fluid decreased
_____ c. Potassium increased
3. Is extracellular fluid excess or deficit diagnosed from the electrolyte report?
_____ Yes
_____ No
4. Accurate daily weights are vital in evaluating extracellular fluid changes.
_____ True
_____ False
5. Changes in blood pressure may indicate extracellular fluid changes.
_____ True
_____ False

**CASE STUDY
2.2**

The emergency room admitted a 59-year-old man who appeared acutely ill.

Signs:. Pale and weak.

Vital signs: Blood pressure (BP) 98/70 (faint), pulse (P) 104 (weak), respiration (R) 44, and temperature (T) 94.

Symptoms: Vomiting four days, weight loss, anorexia, pain in epigastrium, intermittent diarrhea for two weeks.

Shortly after admission, the patient vomited "coffee-ground material" which also contained what appeared to be fresh blood. The patient mentioned to the nurse that he had not voided for four days. There was no bladder distention or discomfort at this time. Laboratory reports:

Serum electrolytes: Na 121 mEq/L; K 4.6 mEq/L; Cl 82 mEq/L; CO_2 9 mEq/L; BUN 139 mg %.

Hematology: HCT 57%; **Hgb** 18.8 gm; WBC 23,600 cu mm; RBC 6,780,000 cu mm.

Questions

1. List the signs and symptoms that suggest fluid and electrolyte imbalance. With what specific imbalance are these associated?

---

*For answers to Quizzes, see Appendix 5.

2. Approximately how much sodium (Na^+) and chloride (Cl^-) are lost per liter in vomitus and diarrheic stools?

3. List and evaluate the abnormal fluid and electrolyte laboratory values.

4. Does the hematology report indicate a considerable blood loss?

5. List the nursing measures that can be initiated immediately.

6. What type of intravenous fluids do you think the physician ordered? Why?

Case Summary: Following rapid, proper treatment and nursing care, this patient was dismissed in four weeks with normal laboratory values. The diagnosis was prerenal failure, extracellular fluid deficit, intracellular fluid excess, renal metabolic acidosis, and gastritis with hemorrhage.

Quiz 2.2

An acutely ill 59-year-old man was admitted to the emergency room with a history of diarrhea, vomiting, weight loss, anorexia, and epigastric pain. He had not voided for four days.
1. Evaluate the extracellular fluid status of this patient upon admission:
   _____ a. Decreased
   _____ b. Normal
   _____ c. Increased
2. Which electrolyte report will tell you that a patient has an extracellular fluid deficit?
   _____ a. Potassium
   _____ b. Serum sodium
   _____ c. None

3. Postural blood pressure and daily weights are valuable aids in determining extracellular fluid deficit.

_____ True

_____ False

4. What is oliguria?

_____ a. Profuse diaphoresis

_____ b. Urine output less than 20 cc/hr, 160 cc/8 hrs, 480 cc/24 hrs

_____ c. Increased excretion of urine

5. Oliguria develops in severe cases of extracellular fluid deficit.

_____ True

_____ False

6. Severe extracellular fluid deficit, with or without hemorrhage, can lead to shock.

_____ True

_____ False

BIBLIOGRAPHY

Abbott Laboratories: Fluid and Electrolytes, Some Practical Guides to Clinical Use, ed. 2. Abbott Laboratories, North Chicago, 1970.

Baxter Laboratories: The Fundamentals of Body Water and Electrolytes. Travenol Laboratories, Inc., Morton Grove, Illinois, 1967.

Lee, C. A., Stroot, V. R., and Schaper, C. A.: Extracellular volume imbalance. Am. J. Nurs. 75:888, 1974.

Maxwell, M. H., and Kleeman, C. R.: Clinical Disorders of Fluid and Electrolyte Metabolism, ed. 2. McGraw-Hill Book Company, New York, 1972.

Meltzer, L. E., Abdellah, F. G., and Kitchell, J. R.: Concepts and Practices of Intensive Care for Nurse Specialists. The Charles Press, Philadelphia, 1969.

Metheny, N. M., and Snively, W. D., Jr.: Nurses' Handbook of Fluid Balance, ed. 2. J. B. Lippincott Company, Philadelphia, 1974.

Paton, R.R., Hegstrom, R.M., and Orme, B.M.: Fluid-Electrolyte Disorders. Mason Clinic, Seattle, 1969.

Scribner, B. H., and Burnell, J. M.: The Teaching Syllabus for the Course on Fluid and Electrolyte Balance, ed. 7. University of Washington, Seattle, 1969.

NOTES

NOTES

3

Intracellular Fluid: Excess and Deficit

The **intracellular fluid** compartment is the area within the cell. Unlike the extracellular fluid compartment, the intracellular fluid compartment contains only a trace of sodium chloride. Therefore the fluid within the intracellular fluid compartment is not a saline solution (NaCl). Thus the intracellular fluid compartment is referred to as the water compartment.

Because the body water moves freely across the cell membrane (osmosis) and the solutes do not move as readily, the concentration or osmolarity of the solute will be the same in both the extracellular and the intracellular fluid compartments. Therefore, our concern in discussing intracellular fluid is with the degree of concentration or dilution of solute in the cellular fluid.

Fluid Distribution

Intracellular fluid represents about 40 per cent of the total body weight. A 165-pound (75 kg) man will have approximately 30 liters of intracellular fluid in his body. This is approximately two thirds of the total amount of body fluid. Extracellular fluid constitutes the other one third.

All fluids taken into the body pass into the extracellular fluid; however, since osmosis and diffusion cause free movement of water across the cell membrane, two thirds of this fluid passes into the intracellular fluid compartment, leaving only one third in the extracellular fluid compartment (Fig. 3-1). When water is lost from the body, two thirds of the total amount will be lost from the intracellular fluid compartment and one third lost from the extracellular compartment. As discussed in Chapter 2, the immediate sensible/insensible loss is from the extracellular fluid compartment; however, it must be remembered that the eventual loss is from the intracellular fluid compartment.

Electrolyte Distribution

The major electrolytes of the intracellular fluid **(ICF)** are potassium, magnesium, phosphate, and protein. Figure 3-2 shows the distribution of electrolytes in intracellular fluid. Potassium is the principal cation; phosphate is the principal anion. Excesses or deficits of electrolytes in the intracellular fluid do not seem to change the cell volume. Cell volume is regulated by changes in the amount of total body water.

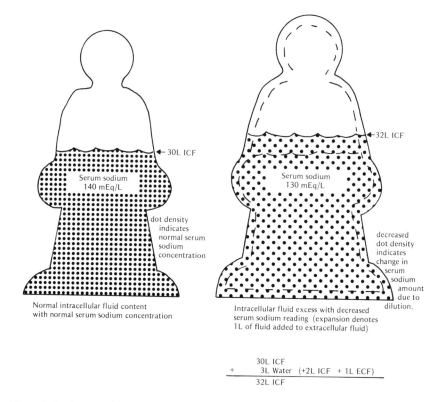

Figure 3-1. Increased intracellular fluid. Three liters of fluid are added to the total body fluid. Note that the intracellular fluid has increased by 2 liters with the remaining 1 liter being distributed to the extracellular fluid. The result is dilution of the serum sodium concentration and a lowered serum sodium reading.

Maintaining Water Balance

There are two main mechanisms for maintaining water balance: the **hypothalmic** thirst center and the **antidiuretic hormone (ADH).** The hypothalmic thirst center is usually activated by a 1 or 2 per cent decrease in the amount of total body water which stimulates the need for water ingestion. The antidiuretic hormone is released by the posterior pituitary gland when there is a need for water. ADH acts on the kidney tubules, causing them to reabsorb water and thereby to correct the water deficit.

INTRACELL-ULAR FLUID EXCESS

Intracellular fluid excess develops when there is an excess of total body water causing the cell volume to increase. As a result, the solute within the cell becomes diluted (see Fig. 3-1).

Causes of Intracellular Fluid Excess

Intracellular fluid excess is most commonly caused by primary renal disease, excessive water intake, or inappropriate ADH secretion. Table 3-1 further explains the causes of the altered functions which result in intracellular fluid excess.

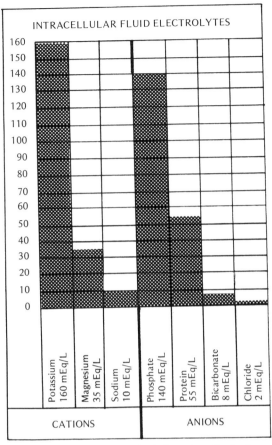

Figure 3-2.   Intracellular fluid electrolyte distribution.

The signs and symptoms displayed by the patient with intracellular fluid excess are exhibited through the central nervous system. These include mental confusion, headache, muscle twitching, coma, and convulsions. The swelling of the cells caused by the excess intracellular fluid leads to increased intracranial pressure (cerebral edema). Peripheral edema would cause the brain cells to swell, rupture, and cause death before the edema would be apparent.

Accurate charting can help the nurse recognize intracellular fluid excess. Both body weight and blood pressure may increase. Urinary output will decrease. This decrease may lead to oliguria.

The best indicator of intracellular fluid disorders is the serum sodium electrolyte test (see Fig. 3.1). This test can verify the nurse's observations of signs and symptoms indicative of intracellular fluid excess. Many nurses incorrectly interpret the serum sodium test as an indication of extracellular fluid disorders; however, this test is *only* applicable to intracellular fluid disorders. When the serum sodium level is below 130 mEq/L, it indicates an

TABLE 3-1. CAUSES OF INTRACELLULAR FLUID EXCESS

Cause	Altered Function
Primary renal disease	Kidneys unable to excrete the water load
Prerenal conditions	
Cardiac insufficiency	Decreased renal perfusion due to inadequate cardiac pump; thus fluid is retained by the body
Cirrhosis	Decreased hepatic perfusion; decreased renal blood flow
Hypoalbuminemia	Insufficient intravascular protein resulting in movement of saline fluid into interstitial areas
Excessive water intake	Excessive oral intake or too rapid administration of intravenous water solution

Stress mechanism
   Postoperative condition
   Narcotics
	Inappropriate and/or excessive release of ADH causing water retention and water intoxication

Hemorrhage	Blood loss causes thirst; water ingested will not replace blood, will only dilute remaining solute

intracellular fluid excess. The solute in the extracellular fluid is diluted by the excess of water; this dilution (hypo-osmolarity) causes the lowered serum sodium reading.

The nurse should be alert to possible excessive administration of intravenous glucose or Mannitol, as these can dilute the serum sodium, creating the false impression of intracellular fluid excess.

The hematocrit is usually normal because the red blood cells swell in proportion to the increase in plasma volume.

Treatment

The treatment for intracellular fluid excess is to restrict fluid intake and correct the contributing causes.

Nurse's Responsibilities

Maintain accurate intake-output records.

Obtain accurate body weight and blood pressure measurements. (Increases above the baseline can be an indicator that intracellular fluid excess exists.)

Restrict fluids as ordered.

Regulate the rate of administration of intravenous fluids carefully to prevent water excess. Avoid too rapid administration.

Be alert to sensorium changes and to central nervous system symptoms.

Report a serum sodium level of 130 mEq/L or below to the physician; withhold liquids until orders are received.

Be aware of conditions under which intracellular fluid excess is likely to develop.

The nurse must be aware of the fact that he is the primary contact between the patient and his health care program. He must be alert to the patient's signs and symptoms as well as the laboratory test results and be careful in conveying this information to the correct member of the health team.

As shown in Figure 3-3, intracellular fluid deficit occurs when a reduction in the amount of total body water causes the cell volume to decrease and the solute to become concentrated.

Intracellular deficit most commonly occurs when water is unavailable, when the patient cannot swallow, or when the patient loses an excessive amount of water. (See Table 3-2 for expanded listing.)

An intracellular fluid deficit causes the cells to shrink. Shrinkage of brain cells affects the central nervous system. The change in the nervous system causes the patient to experience weakness, restlessness, delirium, tetany, and **hyperpnea,** all of which could be followed by sudden respiratory arrest.

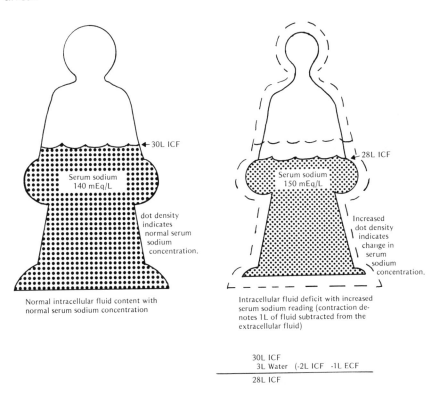

Normal intracellular fluid content with normal serum sodium concentration

Intracellular fluid deficit with increased serum sodium reading (contraction denotes 1L of fluid subtracted from the extracellular fluid)

30L ICF
3L Water (-2L ICF   -1L ECF
28L ICF

Figure 3-3.   Decreased intracellular fluid. Three liters of fluid are subtracted from the total body water. Note that the intracellular fluid decreased by 2 liters with the remaining 1 liter being subtracted from the extracellular fluid. The result is a concentration of the serum sodium content and an elevated serum sodium reading.

TABLE 3-2. CAUSES OF INTRACELLULAR FLUID DEFICIT

Cause	Altered Function
INSUFFICIENT WATER INTAKE	
Confused or comatose condition	Unable to respond to thirst stimulus
Postoperative condition	NPO without sufficient intravenous (IV) maintenance
Desert	Water not available
Inability to swallow	No water ingested; insufficient IV maintenance
High protein tube feeding	Inadequate water instillation between feedings
Diets with increased milk and cream	Insufficient water ingested
EXCESSIVE WATER LOSSES	
Fever and/or diaphoresis	Increased water loss through skin and lungs
Diarrhea	Increased forward peristalsis shortens absorption period
Diabetes insipidus	Increased water loss due to insufficient ADH release
Diabetes mellitus	Insufficient insulin causes hyperglycemia which acts as an osmotic diuretic
Hyperventilation	Excessive insensible water loss due to increased respiration
Prolonged use of artificial respirator	Excessive water loss with administration of dehumidified oxygen

The skin of the patient with intracellular fluid deficit is flushed, and his temperature is elevated. Oliguria occurs as intracellular fluid deficit progresses.

Laboratory Tests

The serum sodium test, an indicator for intracellular fluid excess, is also an indicator for intracellular fluid deficit. A serum sodium level above 145 mEq/L indicates an intracellular fluid deficit. The patient's plasma protein and urinary specific gravity are elevated.

Treatment

The treatment for intracellular fluid deficit is to replace the water either by oral means or by intravenous infusion of 5 per cent dextrose in distilled water and, of course, to correct the underlying cause.

Nurse's Responsibilities

Maintain accurate intake-output records.
Measure and record all liquid stools.

Measure and record accurate body weights.

Be alert to sensorium changes and central nervous system signs and symptoms.

Report a serum sodium level over 145 mEq/L to the physician.

Administer fluids as ordered and encourage patients whose temperature is elevated to drink fluids.

Be especially conscientious in assisting patients who cannot or will not drink fluids.

It is not unusual for a patient to be in a water-depleted condition upon admission to the health care facility. The professional nurse interviews every patient upon admission, records his observations, and takes action as indicated. This is a responsibility of the professional level of nursing because it involves assessing the patient's baseline status. Intracellular fluid deficit can often be prevented by the nurse who is alert to its predisposing conditions.

CASE STUDY 3.1*

Following an illness of three weeks duration, a 60-year-old woman was hospitalized with the following signs and symptoms:

Signs: generalized body weakness

Vital signs: Blood pressure (BP) 160/80; pulse (P) 80; respiration (R) 24; temperature (T) 98.

Symptoms: headache, nausea, vomiting, persistent pain across the upper mid-abdomen, 10-pound weight loss

Patient states she is being hospitalized for X rays and blood tests for possible peptic ulcer, small bowel obstruction, or pancreatitis.

Discussion Questions

1. List the signs and symptoms that are suggestive of fluid and electrolyte imbalance(s). With what specific imbalance are these associated?

2. The admission urinalysis indicated 10-15 WBC/**HPF.** The CBC results were as follows: RBC 3,650,000 cu mm; WBC 6,900 cu mm; HGB 10.1 gm%; HCT 31%; BUN 40 mg%. Evaluate abnormal CBC.

3. Three days following the admission urinalysis report, the physician ordered a catheterized urinalysis. The nurse was unable to obtain any urine by catheter, and at this time the patient casually mentioned that she often goes a day or so without voiding. What should the immediate nurse action be with this added information?

---

*For answers to Case Study Questions, see Appendix 4.

4. The physician determined that lack of output was due to poor intake because of nausea and periodic vomiting. Patient was placed on an IV regime. Two days later patient was still unable to void. Stat electrolyte report results were as follows: BUN 80 mg%; Na 121 mEq/L; K 4 mEq/L; Cl 84 mEq/L; CO_2 14 mEq/L. List and evaluate the abnormal electrolyte values.

5. The next day a cystoscopy revealed a bilateral ureteral obstruction. Ureteral catheters were inserted. The patient's urinary output over the next 24 hours was 8,940 cc with a 4,100 cc intake. Electrolyte report: Na 142 mEq/L; K 3.4 mEq/L: Cl 108 mEq/L: CO_2 22 mEq/L; BUN 30 mg%. Is there a potential problem with an output of 8,940 cc?

6. What do the fall in BUN and the rise in CO_2 indicate?

Case summary: A permanent nephrostomy was performed and the patient was dismissed after normal electrolyte and BUN test results were obtained.

Quiz 3.1*

Following an illness of three weeks duration, a 60 year-old woman was hospitalized with the following signs and symptoms: generalized body weakness, headache, nausea, vomiting, persistent pain across the upper mid-abdomen, 10-pound weight loss.
1. Vomiting causes loss of Na^+, Cl^-, and K^+. Fill in the blanks of these losses per liter of vomitus:
   Na^+:_____ mEq/L; Cl^-:_____mEq/L; K^+:_____mEq/L.
2. This patient gave a history of drinking very little fluid and frequently not voiding for a day or two. Considering this history, the nurse can assume the patient did not void because of poor fluid intake.
   _____ True
   _____ False
3. Following the release of bilateral ureteral obstruction, the patient had an 8,940 cc output in the next 24 hours. Diuresis can cause serious fluid and electrolyte imbalances.
   _____ True
   _____ False
4. A serum sodium level of 121 indicates _____.

*For answers to Quizzes, see Appendix 5.

A 79-year-old woman was admitted to the hospital from a nursing home. She appeared malnourished, weak, and extremely restless. Her skin was flushed and her sensorium dulled. Her temperature was 101.4 F°, pulse 90, respirations 28, and blood pressure 136/80.

Admission orders:
  Chest X ray
  EKG
  Electrolytes stat
  1000 cc 5% dextrose in a normal saline solution with 30 mEq KCl every 12
    hours
  Diet as tolerated

Questions

1. List possible fluid/electrolyte imbalance(s) based on your clinical observations.

2. Match signs and symptoms with suspected fluid/electrolyte imbalance(s).

3. Electrolyte test report: Na 162 mEq/L; K 2.8 mEq/L; Cl 116 mEq/L; CO_2 28 mEq/L; BUN 90 mg%. List the abnormal electrolytes.

4. Does the serum electrolyte report support your answer to Question 1?

5. What immediate actions should the nurse take upon receiving the electrolyte report?

6. Why is the BUN elevated?

Case Summary: Following notification of the electrolyte report, the physician changed the IV order to 5 per cent dextrose in distilled water with KCl until the electrolytes returned to normal. The patient's condition improved, and she returned to the nursing home.

Quiz 3.2

A 79-year-old woman was admitted to the hospital appearing malnourished, weak, extremely restless, with skin flushed, and sensorium dulled. Serum electrolyte report: Na 162 mEq/L; K 2.8 mEq/L; Cl 116 mEq/L; CO_2 28 mEq/L; BUN 90 mg %.

1. Evaluate:

	Normal	Decreased	Increased
Water:	_____	_____	_____
Saline:	_____	_____	_____
Potassium:	_____	_____	_____
BUN:	_____	_____	_____

2. Which electrolyte test is an indicator of water excess or water deficit?
3. What is the treatment for intracellular deficit?
4. Brain cells shrink in water deficit and cause sensorium changes.
   _____ True
   _____ False
5. Severe water deficit could cause a sudden respiratory arrest.
   _____ True
   _____ False

BIBLIOGRAPHY

Abbott Laboratories: Fluid and Electrolytes, Some Practical Guides to Clinical Use, ed. 2. Abbott Laboratories, North Chicago, 1970.

Baxter Laboratories: The Fundamentals of Body Water and Electrolytes. Travenol Laboratories, Inc., Morton Grove, Illinois, 1967.

Bondy, P. K., and Rosenburg, L. E. (eds.): Duncan's Diseases of Metabolism, ed. 7. W. B. Saunders Company, Philadelphia, 1974.

Kleeman, C. R., and Fichman, M. P.: The clinical physiology of water metabolism. N. Engl. J. Med. 277:1300, 1967.

Harvey, A. McG., and Johns, R. J.: The Principles and Practice of Medicine, ed. 18. Appleton-Century-Crofts Medical, New York, 1972.

Medical Clinics of North America. Vol. 53, No. 2, pp. 412-415. W. B. Saunders Company, Philadelphia, March, 1969.

Meltzer, L. E., Abdellah, F. G., and Kitchell, J. R.: Concepts and Practices of Intensive Care for Nurse Specialists. The Charles Press, Philadelphia, 1969.

Metheny, N. M., and Snively, W. D., Jr.: Nurses' Handbook of Fluid Balance, ed. 2. J. B. Lippincott Company, Philadelphia, 1974.

Paton, R. R., Hegstrom, R. M., and Orme, B. M.: Fluid-Electrolyte Disorders. Mason Clinic, Seattle, 1969.

Pitts, R. F.: Physiology of the Kidney and Body Fluids, ed. 3. Year Book Medical Publishers, Chicago, 1974.

Price, J. D. E., and Lauerner, R. W.: Serum urine osmolalities in the differential diagnosis of polyuric states. J. Clin. Endocrinol. Metab. 26:143, 1966.

Sawyer, R. B., et al.: Hypernatremia with pharmacological doses of steriods. Am. J. Surg. 114:691, 1967.

Scribner, B. H. and Burnell, J. M.: Teaching Syllabus for the Course on Fluid and Electrolyte Balance, ed. 7. University of Washington, Seattle, 1969.

Strauss, M. B.: Body Water in Man. Little, Brown and Company, Boston, 1957.

Wesson, L. G.: Physiology of the Human Kidney. Grune and Stratton, Inc., New York, 1969.

38

NOTES

4

Intracellular and Extracellular Fluids: Combined Problems and Comparative Analysis

It is not uncommon for a patient to develop more than one fluid and electrolyte imbalance at a time. When a combined extracellular fluid (saline) and intracellular fluid (water) imbalance occurs, it is essential that the disorders be recognized as *combined* problems but that each disorder be treated *separately.* Since the nurse may play a greater part in recognition than in treatment, he should review Chapters 2 and 3 whenever a combined problem is suspected.

In extracellular fluid (saline) disorders, the extracellular compartment either *contracts* or *expands,* depending on whether there is a deficit or an excess. There is no electrolyte test for extracellular fluid (saline) problems. In intracellular fluid (water) disorders, the problem lies in the *concentration* or *dilution* of the fluid. The serum sodium test is the electrolyte test for intracellular fluid (water) problems.

Two frequent, misunderstood conditions are an extracellular fluid (saline) deficit with an intracellular fluid (water) excess, and an extracellular fluid (saline) excess with an intracellular fluid (water) excess. Table 4-1 gives examples of combined fluid imbalances. In this condition, the extracellular fluid (saline) compartment has become contracted; while the cells composing the intracellular fluid (water) compartment have become swollen.

Extracellular Deficit and Intracellular Excess

The extracellular fluid deficit is commonly caused by gastrointestinal losses, diaphoresis, or diuretics. When these losses are severe, oliguria develops. Oliguria is caused by decreased renal blood flow **(perfusion)** due to hypovolemia. There is also an increase in the antidiuretic hormone output. The intracellular fluid excess develops when the free water intake is greater than obligatory losses.

With the combined problems of extracellular fluid (saline) deficit and intracellular fluid (water) excess, the low serum sodium level often leads to an incorrect diagnosis and treatment. Scribner states: ''Although it would seem logical to relate serum sodium to sodium need, the relationship gives erroneous information most of the time.''* It is vital to satisfactory treatment that a

---

*Belding H. Scribner and J. M. Burnell: Teaching Syllabus for The Course on Fluid and Electrolyte Balance, ed. 7. University of Washington, Seattle, 1969, p. 43.

TABLE 4-1. EXAMPLES OF COMBINED FLUID PROBLEMS

Problem	Serum Reading mEq/L	Common Cause	Recognition
ECF (SALINE) DEFICIT	Serum sodium 140 (normal)	GI losses	Signs and symptoms
Combined with: ICF (water) deficit	Serum sodium >145 (high)	GI losses; lack of water intake	Signs and symptoms; serum sodium reading
ICF (water) excess	Serum sodium <130 (low)	Water intake with inadequate excretion due to renal deficit	Signs and symptoms; serum sodium reading
ECF (SALINE) EXCESS	Serum sodium 140 (normal)	Congestive heart failure	Edema
Combined with: ICF (water) deficit	Serum sodium >145 (high)	Decrease or lack of water intake	Edema; serum sodium reading
ICF (water) excess	Serum sodium <130 (low)	Water retention due to ECF excess	Edema; serum sodium reading

low serum sodium level be regarded only as evidence of intracellular fluid excess and that the extracellular fluid deficit be diagnosed primarily from the signs and symptoms exhibited by the patient. In this condition, the extracellular fluid (saline) compartment has become expanded and the cells in the intracellular fluid (water) compartment have become swollen.

Extracellular Excess and Intracellular Excess

The causes of extracellular fluid excess were discussed in Chapter 2. Extracellular fluid (saline) excess causes the patient to become edematous. As the underlying disease process becomes severe, the patient often retains water, because the excessive sodium in the extracellular fluid draws free water into the extracellular fluid compartment. In other words, "water goes where the salt is."

In general, hypertonic sodium solutions have no place in the treatment of this combined disorder.

The intracellular fluid (water) excess indicated by the low serum sodium level should be treated with water restriction. The extracellular fluid (saline) excess should be diagnosed and treated as indicated by the signs and symptoms. Unfortunately, "the development of [intracellular fluid] water excess in an edematous patient indicates an almost hopeless prognosis unless the underlying disease can be successfully treated."*

COMPARATIVE ANALYSIS:
INTRACELLULAR VS. EXTRACELLULAR FLUID
EXCESSES AND DEFICITS

	EXTRACELLULAR (SALINE)	INTRACELLULAR (WATER)
DISTRIBUTION:	20% of the total body weight; 1/3 of the total body fluid; approximately 15 L of fluid in a 165-pound (75 kg) man	40% of the total body weight; 2/3 of the total body fluid; approximately 30 L of fluid in a 165-pound (75 kg) man
AREA:	Interstitial and intravascular	Within the cells
EXCESS:	Compartment expanded	Solute diluted
DEFICIT:	Compartment contracted	Solute concentrated
FLUID MOVEMENT:	Saline solutions taken into the body remain in the ECF compartment.	Water solutions taken into the body distribute, with 1/3 going into the ECF compartment and 2/3 going into the ICF compartment
	Saline losses are from the ECF compartment.	Water losses are from both compartments in the proportions stated above.
MAJOR ELECTROLYTES:	Sodium (Na^+), chloride (Cl^-), bicarbonate (HCO_3^-), proteinates	Potassium (K^+), magnesium (Mg^{+2}), phosphates (HPO_4^{-2}), protein
SENSIBLE AND INSENSIBLE LOSSES:	Immediate loss from the ECF	Eventual loss from the ICF
CAUSES OF EXCESSES:	Cardiac insufficiency; cirrhosis; ascites; protein depletion; intravenous saline solutions administered too rapidly; secretion of aldosterone (third factor in stress situations and steroid therapy); nephrosis	Primary renal disease; prerenal conditions; excessive water intake (oral or intravenous); inappropriate ADH secretion; hemorrhage

RECOGNITION OF EXCESSES:	Pitting edema; excessive weight gain; elevated blood pressure; dyspnea; increased fullness of neck veins	Central nervous system symptoms; oliguria
LABORATORY TESTS IN EXCESSES:	No electrolyte report to indicate ECF excess; hematocrit is normal or low (usually low); urine sodium may be low; central venous pressure is normal or elevated	Serum sodium lowered (below 130 mEq/L)
TREATMENT OF EXCESSES:	Diuretics; restriction of sodium and fluid intakes; treatment of underlying disease	Restriction of water intake
CAUSES OF DEFICITS:	Gastrointestinal suction; vomiting; diarrhea; fistulous drainage; diuretics; diaphoresis; excessive tap water enemas, especially in infants	Water not available; inability to swallow; high protein tube feedings with insufficient water intake; excessive water losses
RECOGNITION OF DEFICITS:	Postural blood pressure changes; poor skin turgor; decreased fullness of neck veins; vomiting, weakness, anorexia, and nausea; oliguria	CNS symptoms; flushed skin; elevated temperature; oliguria
LABORATORY TESTS IN DEFICITS:	No electrolyte report to indicate deficit; hematocrit is elevated; urine sodium is decreased; protein is elevated	Serum sodium is elevated (above 145 mEq/L); hematocrit is high or normal; urinary specific gravity is elevated; plasma protein is elevated
TREATMENT OF DEFICITS:	Replacement of fluid with saline solution; correction of causes contributing to losses	Replacement of water orally or intravenously by 5% dextrose in distilled water; correction of underlying cause

A 70-year-old woman was admitted to the hospital with a fractured wrist following a fall at her home. The nursing assessment revealed a long history of hypertension and several episodes of congestive heart failure. The patient was proud of having adhered very strictly to her doctor's orders. She stated that she never strayed from her low sodium diet and took her pills faithfully. Her medication consisted of Aldactone and a potent thiazide diuretic.

The nurse noticed that the patient had poor skin turgor and that her postural blood pressure was 130/74 (supine) and 112/60 (standing). Admission weight was 130 pounds. Patient stated this was 15 pounds below her normal weight. The physician ordered an immediate electrolyte test; the results were as follows: Na 114 mEq/L; Cl 72 mEq/L; K 2.4 mEq/L; CO_2 18 mEq/L; BUN 60 mg %.

The patient was unable to void following admission and the next morning appeared to be confused.

Questions

1. Evaluate the postural blood pressure.

2. Evaluate the electrolyte test results and explain.

Case Summary: This patient was immediately taken off the salt-restricted diet and the diuretics were discontinued. She was treated with normal saline and KCl intravenously for the hypovolemia (ECF deficit) and potassium deficit, respectively. NPO for fluids was ordered to correct the water excess. An adequate urinary output followed correction of the hypovolemic state, and the electrolytes and BUN levels returned to normal.

Quiz 4†

A 70-year-old woman was admitted to the hospital with a fractured wrist. She had a long history of hypertension and episodes of congestive heart failure. She was on a low sodium diet and was taking two diuretics. She had an 18 point drop in systolic pressure when postural blood pressures were taken. Following admission she became oliguric and confused.

Laboratory report: Na 114 mEq/L; Cl 72 mEq/L; K 2.4 mEq/L; CO_2 18 mEq/L; BUN 60 mg %.

1. Check the immediate nurse responsibilities following return of the SMA 6.
_____ a. take daily weight
_____ b. force fluids
_____ c. notify physician
_____ d. restrict fluids
_____ e. measure hourly urine output
_____ f. record intake and output
_____ g. observe and record vital signs q 4 hours
(including postural blood pressure)

*For answers to Case Study Questions, see Appendix 4.   †For answers to Quizzes, see Appendix 5.

2. This patient's sensorium changes were probably caused from the
   _____ _____.

3. What causes sensorium changes in this imbalance?

4. Check the following as true or false:

True	False	
_____	_____	a. Serum sodium level can indicate extracellular fluid changes.
_____	_____	b. **Hypokalemia** can cause electrocardiogram changes.
_____	_____	c. Intracellular fluid changes are indicated by the serum sodium level.
_____	_____	d. Accurate daily weight measurement is a reliable guide to extracellular fluid changes.
_____	_____	e. Oliguria is a sign of impending renal failure.

BIBLIOGRAPHY

Scribner, B. H. and Burnell, J. M.: Teaching Syllabus for the Course on Fluid and Electrolyte Balance, ed. 7. University of Washington, Seattle, 1969.

NOTES

NOTES

SECTION III

ELECTROLYTES

5

Potassium

Potassium is the major intracellular electrolyte. It is the principal cation of the cell. Potassium acts as part of the body's buffer system, and serum potassium affects all types of neuromuscular activities.

Distribution in the Body

The total amount of potassium in the body is related to the size of the individual. This proportional variation is due to the fact that potassium makes up a large portion of the muscular tissue. The averages, however, are 3200 mEq in the male and 2200 mEq in the female.

Potassium is distributed throughout the body in the following proportion: intracellular compartment, 98 per cent; extracellular compartment, 2 per cent. Of the 98 per cent found in the intracellular compartment, 70 per cent (or about 3000 mEq) is found in the skeletal muscle and 28 per cent in the liver and red blood cells. The 2 per cent found in the extracellular compartment (about 50 mEq) is represented by the serum potassium reading. A normal serum potassium reading is between 3.5 and 5.5 mEq/L. Measurement of total body potassium is possible using radioisotopes, but the procedure is too expensive and impractical for most purposes.

The normal movement of potassium between the intracellular and extracellular compartments is controlled by the sodium-potassium pump. This pump is an active transport system that moves substances from an area of lower solute concentration to an area of higher concentration. The pump causes the level of potassium to remain higher inside the cell than outside the cell. Conversely, the sodium remains higher outside the cell than inside the cell. (For further explanation of sodium potassium pump see Chapter 6.) Potassium is in a dynamic state; that is, it is constantly moving in and out of the cells according to the body's needs. The process is identified as either pumping or pulling. Both terms are correct.

Intake and Output

Potassium must be ingested daily, as the body has no effective method of storing it. The daily dietary need for potassium is approximately 40 mEq. A normal diet usually contains 60 to 100 mEq/day. Potassium need can be determined by the serum potassium level. The electrocardiogram (EKG) tracing can be used to monitor more serious potassium imbalances. Potassium can be replaced by either oral or parenteral means.

Potassium balance is regulated by the kidneys. Therefore, the major loss of potassium from the body is through the urine. The kidneys do not conserve potassium. Approximately 2.9 mEq of potassium per gram of protein is lost with the excretion of nitrogen waste products through the kidneys. This potassium loss averages 40 mEq per each liter of urine. Nitrogen waste products are the result of cellular metabolism and occur regardless of other loss mechanisms.

There are two basic methods by which the kidneys regulate the potassium balance. In the first, potassium and hydrogen ions compete for exchange with sodium ions in the renal tubules. Urine salt content is adjusted by the distal convoluted tubules of the kidneys. The second method involves the **mineralcorticoid,** aldosterone. Aldosterone, released by the adrenal cortex, regulates the sodium and potassium balance by its effect on the distal convoluted tubules. Aldosterone causes the kidneys to retain sodium, which in turn retains water. In order to retain the sodium, the body excretes potassium ions. This is particularly significant with the release of adrenal hormones in a stress situation, when potassium is lost while sodium and water are retained in order to maintain adequate blood volume.

Some potassium is lost through gastrointestinal losses. There are approximately 5 to 10 mEq of potassium in each liter of gastrointestinal secretions, the loss of which alone will not usually cause a potassium deficit. Although urinary losses alone can cause a potassium deficit, the nurse should be alert to the possibility of a combination of causes.

Functions

Neuromuscular Activity. The degree of concentration of potassium in the intracellular compartment can vary greatly and still remain nontoxic. In the extracellular compartment, however, potassium can easily become dangerous if the serum level fluctuates beyond the range of 3.5 to 5.5 mEq/L. Thus, excess potassium in the extracellular fluid (above 5.5 mEq/L) can become toxic. An excess of potassium in the blood is called **hyperkalemia.** A deficit of potassium in the blood (below 3.5 mEq/L) is called hypokalemia. Since serum potassium affects all types of neuromuscular activity, either an excess or a deficit may affect the myocardium, resulting in **arrhythmias.** Most of the signs and symptoms for hyperkalemia and hypokalemia are related to neuromuscular system changes. However, the level of potassium excess or deficit at which these signs and symptoms become apparent varies from patient to patient.

Acid-Base Balance. Potassium not only affects neuromuscular activity, it also acts as part of the body's buffer system. The serum potassium level rises with acidosis and falls with alkalosis. The body changes the potassium level by drawing hydrogen ions into the cell or pushing them out. In both cases the potassium level changes to compensate for the hydrogen level changes.

Theoretically, in acidosis the body protects itself from the acid state by moving hydrogen ions into the cell. When hydrogen ions move into the cell, potassium ions move out into the serum to make room for the hydrogen ions.

In Figure 5-1 (A), the hydrogen content in the extracellular fluid is high, indicating a state of acidosis. The cells "soak up" hydrogen ions in an attempt to detoxify the extracellular fluid. However, in order to make room for the hydrogen ions, potassium moves out of the cell into the surrounding interstitial fluid and eventually into the intravascular fluid. Consequently, the serum level of potassium becomes elevated. Plasma potassium increases about 0.6 mEq/L for each 0.1 unit fall in blood pH. This elevated potassium

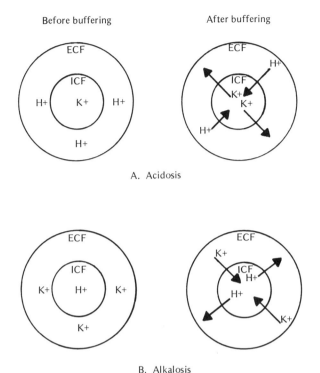

Figure 5-1. Movement of potassium during buffering.

reading is what is called a false positive, since the total body potassium level is not actually elevated. However, potassium above the 5.5. mEq/L level in the serum may become **toxic** regardless of the cause of increase.

As shown in Figure 5-1(B), the opposite is true in the case of alkalosis. In alkalosis, the plasma is low in hydrogen ions. The cells, therefore, release hydrogen ions into the plasma in an attempt to increase the acidity of the blood and combat alkalinity. As a result, potassium moves out of the plasma and into the cells, thereby lowering the serum potassium level. Plasma potassium falls about 0.6 mEq/L for each 0.1 unit rise in blood pH. A level below 3.0 mEq/L is also toxic even though it may be a false negative. A serum reading in this case is also an inaccurate indicator of the total body potassium level since that is unchanged. Nevertheless, both the ''high'' and the ''low'' serum potassium readings are extremely significant because of the potential death-producing consequences of such a shift.

POTASSIUM EXCESS

Potassium balance is one of the most important of electrolyte balances to maintain. Either an excess or a deficit of potassium may cause a crisis situation.

Potassium excess, hyperkalemia, is an increased amount of potassium accumulating in the bloodstream, resulting in a serum potassium reading above 5.5 mEq/L. The major cause of potassium excess is renal disease in which potassium cannot be excreted adequately. It is almost impossible, however, for hyperkalemia to develop when the patient has an adequate urine output. Table 5-1 presents causes and altered functions of potassium excess.

TABLE 5-1. CAUSES OF POTASSIUM EXCESS

Cause	Altered Function
Kidney disease	Potassium retained in the blood; kidneys do not perform proper active transport to eliminate potassium via the collecting tubules into the urine
Rapid IV administration of potassium chloride (KCl)	Potassium administered faster than the kidneys can excrete it
Burns	Increased cellular destruction due to chemical, thermal, or electrical injury releasing potassium from the cell into the extracellular fluid
Crushing injuries	Cellular breakage releasing potassium from the cell into the extracellular fluid
Adrenal insufficiency	Inadequate amounts of glucocorticoid and mineralcorticoid hormones produced causing the body to retain potassium and release too much sodium

Recognition

Because potassium is related to neuromuscular irritability, many of the signs and symptoms of potassium excess stem from the nervous and muscular systems. The signs or symptoms are usually nonspecific. In many cases, clinical signs and symptoms will be absent, so that recognition must often be based on combinations of nonspecific signs and symptoms. Earlier recognition is possible if the patient is on a cardiac monitor, since the cardiac tracings will show very definite and specific changes. These EKG changes include tented T waves, elevated T waves, widened QRS, prolonged P-R interval, flattening to absent P waves, and ST segment depression (see Fig. 5-2).

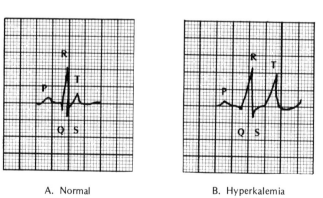

A. Normal   B. Hyperkalemia

Figure 5-2. EKG tracings demonstrating changes which occur with hyperkalemia.

Table 5-2 lists the signs and symptoms presented by the body systems during hyperkalemia.

Death in hyperkalemia usually results when the toxic state causes cardiac arrhythmia (ventricular fibrillation or atrial standstill).

TABLE 5-2. SIGNS AND SYMPTOMS OF POTASSIUM EXCESS

System	Signs and Symptoms
Skeletal	Weakness, flaccid paralysis
Neural	Twitching, **hyperreflexia** proceeding to **paresthesia** and paralysis
Cardiac	Bradycardia proceeding to cardiac arrest (flat P wave – atrial arrest); ventricular fibrillation; cardiac arrest may occur without any warning other than EKG changes
Urinary	Oliguria

Laboratory Tests

The serum potassium level will be over 5.5 mEq/L.

Treatment

The treatment of hyperkalemia will vary according to the severity of the problem. Therapy can include rapid intravenous administration of hypertonic glucose with insulin. The glucose and insulin move into the cell, pulling the potassium with it. Once the potassium is in the cell, it is no longer toxic. This procedure lessens an acute condition until the underlying cause of the hyperkalemia can be corrected or its effect diminished.

Hypertonic Kayexalate may be given orally or as an enema to be retained for a period of time. Kayexalate acts as an exchange resin that absorbs the potassium into the gastrointestinal tract. When Kayexalate is used as an enema, the potassium is evacuated along with the solution. A bulb catheter may be used to hold the solution in the body following instillation.

Since potassium depresses the heart, in emergencies intravenous administration of calcium may also be ordered to stimulate the heart. Calcium should not be administered if the patient is taking a digitalis preparation because the combined treatments may result in cardiac arrhythmias. Examples of such calcium preparations are gluconate and gluceptate.

Peritoneal and hemodialysis are also part of the treatment of acute conditions (see Chapters 20 and 21). By different methods, both procedures filter the potassium and waste products from the extracellular fluid.

A sodium deficiency may also cause hyperkalemia. Increasing the sodium increases the loss of potassium through the kidneys, thereby eliminating the excess.

If necrotic tissue is involved, débridement may be necessary to remove injured and dead cells which are releasing potassium into the vascular system.

Excessive or too rapid administration of potassium may also cause hyperkalemia; in such a case, administration must be discontinued at once. Potassium should never be given in a direct undiluted injection. The average dose is 40 mEq/L, not to be administered faster than 20 mEq/hr unless specifically ordered; in this case, the patient should be monitored.

In hyperkalemic conditions when blood transfusions are ordered to correct other problems, transfuse with fresh blood if possible. Transfusions of stored blood may elevate the potassium level because the breakdown of older blood cells releases potassium.

When hyperkalemia and acidosis exist concurrently, the lactate or bicarbonate used to correct the acidosis will also drive the potassium back into the cells.

Nurse's Responsibilities

Be alert to conditions that can lead to hyperkalemia.
Take preventive measures whenever possible.
Observe for pulse changes and/or EKG changes.
Observe for signs and symptoms of potassium excess.
Check the serum potassium reports; notify physician when potassium is 6 mEq/L or above.
Give fresh blood transfusions if possible.
Do not give calcium if the patient is also taking a digitalis preparation.

POTASSIUM DEFICIT

Potassium deficit, or hypokalemia, is the loss of potassium from the body resulting in a serum potassium reading below 3.5 mEq/L. The major cause of potassium deficit is increased renal loss. A common factor is the use of diuretics. Other factors that contribute to a potassium deficit are insufficient potassium intake, urinary losses (both normal and excessive), and gastrointestinal losses. Although urinary losses alone can cause a potassium deficit, the nurse should be alert to a possible combination of causes. Table 5-3 lists the causes and altered functions of potassium deficit.

TABLE 5-3. CAUSES OF POTASSIUM DEFICIT

Cause	Altered Function
RENAL LOSSES	
Potassium-losing nephritis	Kidneys retain sodium chloride and lose potassium
Renal tubular acidosis	Tubular dysfunction causes loss of fluids and electrolytes
Diuretic phase of acute renal failure - Diuretic therapy (especially thiazide group)- Healing stage of burns	Potassium lost in proportion to amount of diuresis
Diabetic acidosis	Hyperglycemia causes diuresis resulting in potassium loss
Cushing's syndrome - Corticosteroid therapy	Hormonal imbalance causes sodium and chloride retention and potassium loss
INADEQUATE INTAKE	
Starvation	Lack of potassium intake and additional loss due to stress response
Potassium-free intravenous therapy	Prolonged potassium-free IV fluids combined with no food intake
Low sodium diet	When salt substitute containing potassium is not consumed, insufficient potassium intake results

TABLE 5-3. (continued)

GASTROINTESTINAL LOSSES

Gastrointestinal suction	Evacuation of ECF containing potassium by mechanical means, such as Levin or Cantor tubes
Fistulas	Tubelike passageway between the GI tract and an external surface allows ECF and potassium loss
Vomiting	Reversed peristalsis causes loss of extracellular secretions containing potassium
Diarrhea - Chronic laxative abuse	Increased forward peristalsis shortens absorption period and prevents absorption of potassium

ACID-BASE IMBALANCE

Alkalosis	Serum potassium may be low due to shift of potassium into cell as hydrogen moves out of cell in an attempt to correct the alkalosis.
Acidosis	In acidosis a normal serum potassium reading indicates potassium deficit, since acidosis should cause a high potassium reading. Treat the potassium deficit as the acidosis is corrected.

Recognition

In hypokalemia, as well as in hyperkalemia, many of the signs and symptoms originate in the nervous and muscular systems and are usually nonspecific. Muscular weakness and fatigue are early signs noted by the patient. Another early sign is a change in the EKG. These changes include peaking of P waves, flat T waves, depressed S-T segments, and elevated U waves (see Fig. 5-3).

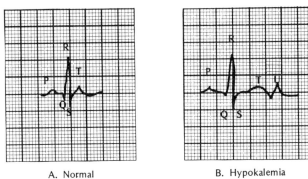

A. Normal   B. Hypokalemia

Figure 5-3.   EKG tracings demonstrating changes which occur with hypokalemia.

Table 5-4 lists signs and symptoms of potassium deficit and the affected body system.

TABLE 5-4. SIGNS AND SYMPTOMS OF POTASSIUM DEFICIT

System	Signs and Symptoms
Skeletal	Muscle weakness, muscle pain, flabby muscles, fatigue, hyporeflexia
Cardiac	Hypotension (decreased stroke volume), arrhythmias, enhanced digitalis intoxication. (Note: Digitalis, diuretics, and hypokalemia are a potentially lethal combination.)
Respiratory	Respiratory muscle weakness procceding to paralysis; cyanosis and eventual respiratory arrest
Gastrointestinal	Anorexia proceeding to nausea, vomiting, and paralytic ileus
Neural	Apathy, drowsiness, irritability, paresthesia, tetany, coma

In hypokalemia, death usually is caused by the anoxia created by the paralysis of the respiratory muscles, leading to a cardiac arrest.

Recognition of hypokalemia in severe acidosis may be difficult because the serum potassium reading will be normal even though a deficit exists. If the serum reading is low during acidosis, a very serious potassium deficit exists.

Laboratory Tests

The serum potassium level is below 3.5 mEq/L.

Treatment

The prevention of conditions predisposed to creating a potassium deficit is the primary objective in regard to hypokalemia. For example, the potassium level should be checked frequently when potent diuretics, particularly the thiazides and the mercurials, are being administered. When a patient is allowed nothing by mouth after surgery, he should receive at least a minimal maintenance dose of potassium in his intravenous fluid plus additional amounts to compensate for loss via other means.

If potassium loss cannot be prevented, then the potassium must be replaced. Potassium can be administered orally as a liquid or tablet. A commonly administered form of potassium is potassium chloride (KCl). In many cases, the patient's chloride level is low when potassium is lost. Other drugs are Kaon and K-Triplex, neither of which is high in chloride. Salt substitutes containing potassium can be part of the treatment plan.

Small bowel lesions may occur due to the ingestion of potassium. Oral administration of potassium may need to be discontinued should any of the following symptoms occur: abdominal pain, distention, nausea, vomiting, or gastrointestinal bleeding. Report these symptoms to the physician.

Lost potassium can be replaced through the diet if the patient is allowed to take fluids and foods orally. Some substances high in potassium content are meat, bananas, orange juice, coffee, tea, cola beverages, and chocolate.

Potassium can also be administered intravenously. Before intravenous administration, however, the patient should be checked for sufficient renal output, since the main outlet for potassium from the body is through the kidneys. If the kidneys are not working properly, a potassium excess could be induced. Only 40 mEq/liter at the rate of 20 mEq/hr or less may be administered safely unless the patient is on a cardiac monitor. A burning sensation at the site of administration may indicate that the concentration is toxic to this particular individual, and thus the fluid administration should be slower.

Aldactone is a diuretic that may be used in congestive heart failure when it is necessary to keep the potassium loss to a minimum. The more potent diuretics (thiazides especially) cause the loss of sodium, chloride, and potassium; therefore, as their use may cause or enhance a potassium deficit, it should be carefully evaluated by the physician.

Nurse's Responsibilities

Since the primary objective is prevention of hypokalemia, be alert to conditions that cause potassium loss.

Maintain accurate intake-output records to aid physician in calculating potassium replacement need.

Observe for pulse (tachycardia) and/or EKG changes.

Check serum potassium reports; notify physician when potassium is 3 mEq/L or below.

Administer oral potassium preparations with at least four ounces of water to prevent gastrointestinal irritation.

Observe for signs of metabolic alkalosis (see Chapter 10 for a thorough discussion).

Be alert to patients receiving digitalis and diuretics, as cardiac arrhythmia can occur if hypokalemia develops.

Remember that hypokalemia enhances the effect of digitalis, creating the possibility of digitalis intoxication from even an average maintenance dose.

The physician will estimate the total body loss of potassium from the observations and figures the nurse supplies. From this he will determine the amount and method of replacement (oral, intravenous, or dietary). Usually one half of the total loss is replaced in the first 24 hours. If more rapid replacement is needed, the patient must be carefully monitored because of the danger of potassium-induced arrhythmias. Use of micro- and minidrop meters on the intravenous tubing facilitates counting the drops of intravenous fluid more accurately.

Although the symptoms for hyperkalemia and hypokalemia are similar and nonspecific, they should alert the nurse to take appropriate, immediate action.

CASE STUDY 5.1*

A 20-year-old girl was admitted to the hospital following a car-train collision. She appeared to have internal injuries and was thought to be hemorrhaging. She remained hypotensive throughout emergency surgery for removal of a ruptured spleen. Following surgery and blood transfusions her condition remained stable for four days. Urine output then began decreasing, while BUN and serum potassium levels showed elevation.

Questions

1. Discuss the relationship between decreased urinary output and elevation of BUN and serum potassium levels.

---

*For answers to Case Study Questions, see Appendix 4.

2. The urinary output continued to decrease, and the patient became oliguric. It was determined that she had developed an acute renal failure and should be placed on hemodialysis (artificial kidney) for six-hour periods. This procedure was tolerated well, but the elevation of the serum potassium level continued to be a major problem between dialyses. Was there a specific reason for the difficulty in controlling the serum potassium between dialyses?

3. Several days after hemodialysis was started, the serum potassium report was returned to the nursing unit reading 7.7 mEq/L. The nurse on duty did not feel that action was necessary at this time because the patient was to be placed on hemodialysis within an hour. Was the nurse's decision correct?

4. Following persistent urging from another nurse, the physician was called. He ordered 300 cc Na lactate, 50 cc of 5 per cent glucose with 10 units of insulin to be given intravenously immediately. What is the action of this medication?

5. What would you expect to find in the EKG pattern?

Quiz 5.1*

A 20-year-old girl was admitted to the hospital following a car-train accident. Several days after emergency surgery her BUN level was 83 mg % and the serum potassium was 6.3 mEq/L.

1. Evaluate:

BUN:	_____normal	_____increased	_____decreased
Serum K:	_____normal	_____increased	_____decreased

2. Under normal circumstances how does the body maintain a potassium balance?

3. The physician should be notified when the serum potassium level is above_____.

4. In hyperkalemia, cardiac arrest can occur with no warning except EKG changes. _____True _____False

5. Cite three circumstances in which serum potassium could rise above its normal range.

---

*For answers to Quizzes, see Appendix 5.

A 68-year-old woman was admitted to the hospital with a six-week history of diarrhea. She complained of severe muscular weakness. Electrolyte test results were: Na 142 mEq/L; K 1.5 mEq/L; Cl 92 mEq/L; CO_2 32 mEq/L.

Questions

1. Which electrolyte levels are abnormal?

2. What should the immediate nursing action be, and why?

3. What nursing measures should the nurse carry out and what observations should she make without a physician's orders?

4. The physician ordered intravenous fluids with KCl, but did not specify rate of flow. What is the usual amount of flow rate of potassium per liter?

5. When an emergency situation requires both an increased amount of KCl per liter and a more rapid rate of flow, the patient should be placed on a cardiac monitor and a microdrip used. What changes could be expected on the EKG?

Quiz 5.2

A 68-year-old woman was admitted to the hospital with a six-week history of diarrhea. She complained of severe muscular weakness. Electrolyte test results were: Na 142 mEq/L; K 1.5 mEq/L; Cl 92 mEq/L; CO_2 32 mEq/L.
1. Evaluate the following:

	Normal	Decreased	Increased
Saline	_____	_____	_____
Water	_____	_____	_____
Potassium	_____	_____	_____

2. A serum potassium level of 1.5 is a medical emergency.
_____ True _____ False

3. The greatest danger for this patient was:
   _____ a. falling from weakness;
   _____ b. respiratory paralysis leading to arrhythmia;
   _____ c. development of hypertension.
4. Should this patient be given direct intravenous injections of KCl?

5. The physician should be notified when the serum potassium level is below _____.

BIBLIOGRAPHY

American Hospital Formulary Service. American Society of Hospital Pharmacists, Washington, 1972.

Berlinger, R. W.: Renal mechanisms for potassium excretion. Harvard Lect. 55:141, 1961.

Brooks, S. M.: Basic Facts of Body Water and Ions, ed. 3. Springer Publishing Company, New York, 1973.

Dutcher, I. E. and Fielo, S. B.: Water and Electrolytes: Implications for Nursing Practice. The Macmillan Company, New York, 1967.

Goldberger, E.: A Primer of Water, Electrolyte and Acid-Base Syndromes, ed. 5. Lea and Febiger, Philadelphia, 1975.

Harvey, A. McG., and Johns, R. J.: The Principles and Practice of Medicine, ed. 18. Appleton-Century-Crofts Medical, New York, 1972.

Janz, G. J., and Tomkins, R. P. T.: Nonaqueous Electrolyte Handbook, ed. 2. Academic Press, New York, 1973.

Krupp, M. A., et al.: Physician's Handbook, ed. 17. Lange Medical Publications, Los Altos, California, 1973.

Metheny, N. M. and Snively, W. D., Jr.: Nurses' Handbook of Fluid Balance, ed. 2. J. B. Lippincott, Philadelphia, 1974.

Paton, R. R., Hegstrom, R. M., and Orme, B. M.: Fluid-Electrolyte Disorders. Mason Clinic, Seattle, 1969.

Pitts, R. F.: Physiology of the Kidney and Body Fluids, ed. 3. Year Book Medical Publishers, Inc. Chicago, 1974.

Rosenfeld, M. G. (ed.): Manual of Medical Therapeutics, ed. 20. Little, Brown and Company, Boston, 1971.

Schwartz, W. B., Van Ypersele de Strihou, C., and Kassirer, J. P.: Medical progress: Role of anions in metabolic alkalosis and potassium deficiency. N. Engl. J. Med. 279:630, 1968.

Scribner, B. H. and Burnell, J. M.: Teaching Syllabus for the Course of Fluid and Electrolyte Balance, ed. 7. University of Washington, Seattle, 1969.

Snipes, R.: Statistical Mechanical Theory of the Electrolytic Transport of Non-electrolytes. Springer-Verlag Inc., New York, 1973.

Steinmetz, P. R., and Kiley, J. E.: Hypercalcemia in renal failure. J.A.M.A. 175:689, 1961.

Wesson, L. G.: Physiology of the Human Kidney. Grune and Stratton, Inc., New York, 1969.

NOTES

NOTES

6

Sodium

Sodium is the major component of the extracellular saline solution. The combination of sodium and chloride in water constitutes a saline solution. Sodium and chloride balances may become deranged independently of each other. A sodium imbalance can result from a loss or gain of sodium or a change in water volume. A change in the combination of the electrolytes (sodium and chloride) also causes a change in the water quantity of the extracellular fluid, as both tend to hold water (see Chapter 4).

Three factors can create a sodium imbalance. One is a change in the sodium content of the extracellular fluid, such as a deficit due to excessive vomiting or an excess due to a failure to excrete sodium. The second is a change in the chloride content which can affect both the sodium concentration and the amount of water in the extracellular fluid. When the chloride is out of proportion to the sodium, it is reflected in an acid-base imbalance. The third factor is a change in the quantity of water in the extracellular fluid. Because only one third of the total body fluid is extracellular, a serum sodium change indicates the major problem is a total body water imbalance.

Sodium, because it is part of the composition of the extracellular fluid, affects the distribution of electrolytes in this compartment. However, one of the major characteristics of sodium is its ability to attract water, and because any alteration in the water level of the body affects primarily the intracellular area, any alteration in the serum sodium level should be considered an *intracellular* rather than an extracellular problem. The effect of sodium on the body is analogous to that of a pebble dropped into a pond. The pebble affects its immediate surroundings (the extracellular compartment) only slightly, whereas the shock waves created by the pebble wash across the pond and have a proportionately greater effect on the beach (the intracellular compartment).

The average adult consumes approximately six grams of sodium per day. The minimum daily sodium need, with no excess losses, is two grams. The most common source of sodium is sodium chloride (salt). Sodium is absorbed actively by the intestines and excreted through the kidneys and skin.

The amount of sodium in the extracellular fluid is controlled by the release of aldosterone through a feedback mechanism that functions in the following way: Aldosterone is secreted by the adrenal cortex and acts upon the renal distal tubules to reabsorb sodium. When sodium is reabsorbed, the sodium content in the extracellular fluid is increased. The increased sodium in the extracellular fluid in turn causes a decrease in the amount of aldosterone secreted. Since the feedback mechanism is a two-way relationship, a decrease in the amount of aldosterone secretion results in an increase in the amount of sodium lost via the urine (see Fig. 6-1).

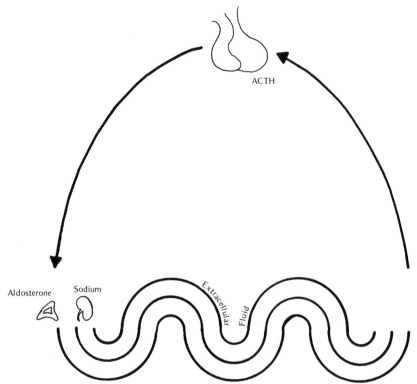

Figure 6-1. Negative feedback mechanism. Decreased sodium in the ECF results in the release of ACTH from the anterior pituitary which causes an increase in aldosterone. Aldosterone in turn causes the retention of sodium.

Distribution in the Body

Sodium is the primary cation in the extracellular fluid. It composes about 90 per cent of the total cation content, which is approximately 142 mEq/L in a normal extracellular fluid concentration.

Functions

Because sodium does not easily penetrate the cell membrane, it is a primary regulator in the relationship of body fluids.

Both sodium and chloride are important factors in the body's ability to retain water. When sodium is reabsorbed, chloride is usually reabsorbed with it. The effect of their combined reabsorption is to increase the amount of water held by the body. Changes in the body fluid level cause corresponding changes in the extracellular fluid volume. Thus the amount of extracellular fluid, both blood volume and interstitial fluid volume, increases as water increases. Sodium changes affect the intracellular fluid as well as the extracellular fluid. Since intracellular fluid represents two thirds and extracellular fluid represents one third of the total amount of body water, all increases or losses of body water are reflected proportionately in each compartment; i.e., by a two-thirds change in the intracellular fluid volume and a one-third change in the extracellular fluid volume. Although sodium changes affect both intracellular and extracellular fluid, the serum sodium reading only pertains to intracellular fluid changes.

By the process of reabsorption, sodium is able to control maintenance of blood volume and interstitial fluid volume, regulate the shift of water between compartments, and influence the excretion of water.

Sodium also helps regulate acid-base balance because it readily combines with chloride and bicarbonate and can, therefore, help maintain the balance between cations and anions. Sodium, in conjunction with potassium, is responsible for maintaining the normal balance of electrolyte composition in intracellular and extracellular fluids by means of an active transport mechanism (the sodium-potassium pump).

The sodium-potassium pump also influences the irritability of nerves and muscles. Sodium is an important factor in nerve conduction. It aids in establishing the potential of nerve membranes to excite charges. A nerve membrane in a relaxed or resting stage has a positive charge outside and a negative charge inside (see Fig. 6-2). When the membrane becomes more permeable, a small number of potassium ions move out of the cell and, simultaneously, a large number of sodium ions move into the cell. The membrane is now depolarized; the outside of that portion of the membrane is now negatively charged. The depolarization is propagated along the nerve cell. This depolarization wave is called the nerve impulse. Repolarization immediately follows depolarization, thus reestablishing the resting stage. This electrolyte change causes the nerve to conduct electrical impulses to the muscle and causes that muscle to contract. Sodium,

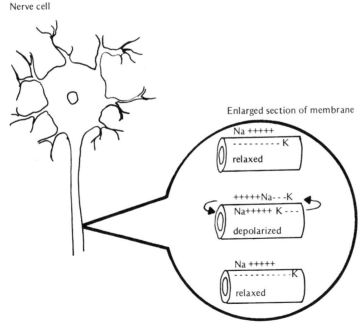

Figure 6-2. Nerve impulse.

therefore, influences the irritability of muscles, nerves, and the heart. Any disturbance in the sodium balance can disturb the synchronization of neuromuscular function.

Hypernatremia

The condition in which there is too much sodium in the serum is called **hypernatremia.** Although *hypernatremia* refers specifically to the sodium concentration in the serum, it is actually a condition of water deficiency resulting in a concentrated or thick serum (see Chapter 3). Figure 6-3 illustrates the concept that the serum sodium reading reflects a change in the *water balance,* not a change in the amount of sodium. Figure 6-3 (B) represents the normal proportional relationship between water and sodium in the serum. (A) shows that when the water in the serum is decreased, the serum sodium reading is increased, even though the amount of sodium remains the same. The reading indicates hypernatremia because the serum is more concentrated. (C) shows that when the water in the serum is increased and the

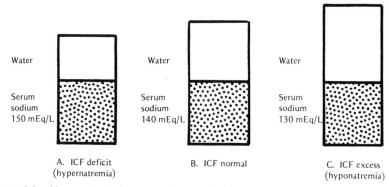

| A. ICF deficit | B. ICF normal | C. ICF excess |
| (hypernatremia) | | (hyponatremia) |

Figure 6-3. Hypernatremia-hyponatremia. Actual sodium content remains the same; only the serum sodium *reading* varies as the ICF level varies.

amount of sodium remains the same, the serum sodium reading is decreased (indicating **hyponatremia**) because the serum has been diluted. The serum sodium concentration can move from a normal of 140 mEq/L to a hypernatremic state of 150 mEq/L by losing water while the mEq of sodium in the body is exactly the same as before the water loss.

Recognition. Recognition of hypernatremia is by the serum sodium level, which is increased with a water deficit. When the actual amount of total body sodium is increased, water is often increased. Thus the signs and symptoms are the same as those of an extracellular fluid excess: pitting edema, excessive weight gain, elevated blood pressure and, in some cases, dyspnea. (These signs and symptoms are discussed in more detail in Chapter 2.)

A hypernatremic state in which the serum sodium reading is increased and water is actually lost will cause the blood to become very concentrated, resulting in dry, sticky mucous membranes, flushed skin, intense thirst, and oliguria. The temperature may become elevated and tachycardia may exist. Death is usually due to an intense rise of osmotic pressure and respiratory arrest. A hypernatremic state may be caused by administering sodium chloride intravenously without replacement of water.

Laboratory Tests. The serum sodium level may be high, low, or normal since this can be a combined problem. If the condition is a saline excess with a water deficit, the serum sodium level will be high. If there is only a saline excess, the serum sodium level may remain unchanged. The specific gravity of the urine will be above 1.030 if there is a water deficit. The urinary sodium level will be decreased. The red blood count and the hematocrit, as well as the serum protein count (blood concentrate), will be elevated.

Hyponatremia

Sodium deficit in the serum is called hyponatremia and is usually caused by excessive sweating, gastrointestinal losses, or the administration of potent diuretics (especially mercurials and thiazides). Deficit may also be related to a lack of sodium intake, adrenal insufficiencies in which sodium cannot be conserved, low salt diets, excessive loss with trauma (especially burns, see Chapter 19), and renal diseases, (see Chapters 14 and 15).

Recognition. If both sodium and water are lost, the signs and symptoms are the same as those listed for an extracellular fluid deficit. These are weakness, restlessness, delirium, hyperpnea, oliguria, elevated temperature, and flushed skin. In addition, the patient may have abdominal cramps and convulsions. A more pronounced or severe deficit can cause vasomotor collapse, such as hypotension, rapid thready pulse, cold clammy skin, and cyanosis. In the early stages of severe deficit, the patient's skin is flushed, but as the patient reaches the shock stage, it becomes cold and clammy.

If sodium is lost and water is not, the signs and symptoms will be the same as those of a water excess. These signs and symptoms are exhibited through the central nervous system: mental confusion, headache, muscle twitching, coma, and convulsions. The patient may also experience lassitude, weakness, giddiness, and syncope on changing position. Blurred vision may also be present. Body weight and blood pressure may stay the same or increase. Urinary output may decrease, leading to oliguria.

Laboratory Tests. The laboratory tests give only an indication, not a direct correlation to what has taken place within the body. If both the sodium and water levels are lowered, there will be no change in the serum sodium reading. A decreased serum sodium level indicates a water excess. If only a saline deficit is present, the serum sodium reading will be normal. When the specific gravity of the urine is decreased (below 1.010), this indicates that the actual sodium in the extracellular fluid concentration is decreased. This test is significant because when sodium is decreased in the body, the kidneys conserve sodium causing less to be present in the urine. In both hypernatremia and hyponatremia, the hematocrit, red blood cell count, and plasma protein reading will be elevated.

Treatment of Sodium Excess and Deficit

Since changes in sodium concentration are reflected by a change in the intracellular or extracellular fluid concentration, treatment is directed towards changing these two variables. If a sodium excess exists in which the sodium and water are both increased, this constitutes an extracellular fluid excess and should be treated as such. The treatment for this type of saline excess is to administer diuretics and restrict the intake of sodium and fluids.

If the signs and symptoms indicate an extracellular fluid deficit, the treatment would usually be the administration of intravenous isotonic or hypertonic saline, depending on the severity of the deficit.

When only the sodium reading is elevated on the serum sodium test, this constitutes an intracellular fluid deficit. The treatment is to replace the water either by oral means or by intravenous infusion of 5 per cent dextrose in distilled water.

If only the sodium reading is decreased on the serum test, this constitutes an intracellular fluid excess. The treatment is to restrict fluid intake.

Nurse's Responsibilities

Condition of Excess:

Observe for fluid volume changes.

Observe for changes in vital signs.

Maintain accurate intake and output records.

Check weight daily.

Check patient history for conditions that may lead to or enhance the problem; e.g., heart disease progressing to congestive heart failure.

Maintain skin and oral care.

Restrict sodium in diet as directed by physician.

Condition of Deficit:

Maintain accurate intake and output records.

Observe for changing signs and symptoms with therapy.

Administer fluids and foods high in sodium as directed by physician.

BIBLIOGRAPHY

Brooks, S. M.: Basic Facts of Body Water and Ions, ed. 3. Springer Publisher Company, New York, 1973.

Goldberger, E.: A Primer of Water, Electrolyte and Acid-Base Syndromes, ed. 5. Lea and Febiger, Philadelphia, 1975.

Harvey, A. McG., and Johns, R. J.: The Principles and Practice of Medicine, ed. 18. Appleton-Century-Crofts Medical, New York, 1972.

Janz, G. J., and Tomkins, R. P. T.: Nonaqueous Electrolyte Handbook, ed. 2. Academic Press, New York, 1973.

Metheny, N. M., and Snively, W. D., Jr.: Nurses' Handbook of Fluid Balance, ed. 2. J. B. Lippincott Company, Philadelphia, 1974.

Scribner, B. H., and Burnell, J. M.: Teaching Syllabus for the Course of Fluid and Elecytrolyte Balance, ed. 7. University of Washington, Seattle, 1969.

NOTES

70

NOTES

7

Chloride

Chloride is the major anion of the extracellular fluid. As was mentioned in the chapter on sodium, chloride varies independently or in relation to sodium and water balances. The combination of sodium and chloride in water composes the saline solution of the extracellular compartment. Both sodium and chloride tend to hold water. Like the serum sodium reading, the serum chloride reading will change as the quantity of extracellular fluid changes (see Fig. 7-1). The exact daily minimum requirement has not been established.

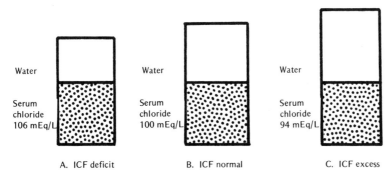

Figure 7-1. Chloride excess-deficit. Actual chloride content remains the same, only the chloride *reading* varies as the ICF level varies.

Distribution in the Body

The normal amount of chloride in the blood is 95 to 105 mEq/L. Chloride is found in greater proportion in the interstitial and lymph fluid compartments. Intracellular chloride is very small in quantity but significant because it is found in certain specialized cells, such as nerve cells.

Functions

Chloride functions, as sodium does, to maintain the osmotic pressure of the blood and thus the blood volume and arterial pressure. Chloride concentration is regulated secondarily to the regulation of sodium concentration. With each sodium ion reabsorbed in the renal tubules, a chloride or bicarbonate ion is also reabsorbed. The amount of chloride or bicarbonate reabsorbed depends on the acid-base balance of the extracellular fluid. (Acid-base balance is discussed in detail in Chapter 9.)

Aldosterone, a mineralcorticoid, indirectly exerts control over the reabsorption of chloride from kidney tubules. As aldosterone causes reabsorption of sodium, chloride is also reabsorbed. Thus the effect of aldosterone is to increase both sodium and chloride (salt) and thus water in the extracellular fluid compartment. When aldosterone holds sodium and chloride, it releases some potassium or hydrogen. The total effect, in which chloride is only one component, is to increase the osmotic pressure of the blood, the total blood volume, and arterial pressure.

Correlation to Sodium Problems

Chloride and sodium usually vary *proportionately* to each other. *However, in metabolic alkalotic states, chloride decreases independently of sodium.*

Chloride is most often associated with sodium and fluid changes. When both the serum chloride and the serum sodium readings are elevated, the recognition, treatment, and nursing responsibilities are the same as those with an intracellular fluid deficit.

A decrease in the chloride and sodium readings correlates with a possible intracellular fluid excess. The recognition, treatment, and nursing responsibilities are the same as those for a water excess.

Correlation to Acid-Base Problems

Chloride Deficit

Because chloride combines with sodium in competition with bicarbonate, it is related to the acid-base balance of the body. Alkalosis may be caused by the loss of a chloride-rich secretion such as the gastric juices. When chloride is decreased, the bicarbonate increases in compensation, because the total anions of the extracellular fluid must always be equal to the total cations in order to preserve acid-base equality. Thus when chloride decreases, extra bicarbonate ions are retained to balance the sodium ions. The result is a **hypochloremic** metabolic alkalosis.

Recognition. Such symptoms as **hypertonicity** of muscles, tetany, and depressed respirations may be present.

Treatment. The primary treatment is to replace the chloride in proportion to the amount which has been lost.

Nurse's Responsibilities. Maintain accurate intake and output records so the physician can calculate the intravenous or oral replacement of chloride with consideration of the possibility of creating a water imbalance.

Observe for respiratory difficulties.

Chloride Excess

Acidosis can be related to an excess of chloride ions being retained or ingested. In this case, with the additional chloride, the bicarbonate ions are released in the kidney tubules, thus lowering the base bicarbonate circulating in the extracellular fluid. This leads to a **hyperchloremic** metabolic acidosis because of the primary deficit in the base bicarbonate concentration in the extracellular fluid.

Recognition. The major signs and symptoms of metabolic acidosis include stupor, deep, rapid breathing, weakness, and in severe acidosis, unconsciousness.

Treatment. The treatment of metabolic acidosis is very complex. In many cases, treatment depends on the underlying cause of the acidosis. These are discussed thoroughly in Chapter 10. However, there are a few general procedures which will be listed here.

In an emergency in which acidity must be reduced rapidly, an intravenous injection of a bicarbonate solution will quickly increase the buffer base of the blood, thereby relieving the acidosis.

In less urgent cases, another intravenous solution which can be used is 5 per cent dextrose in Ringer's lactate solution. This increases the base level of the blood because the liver will convert the sodium lactate to bicarbonate.

The potassium level should be carefully monitored during treatment.

A very thorough understanding of acid-base imbalances is necessary in treating acidosis or alkalosis.

Nurse's Responsibilities. Maintain accurate intake and output records.

Monitor intravenous infusions containing chloride.

Observe for **hyperventilation.**

BIBLIOGRAPHY

Goldberger, E.: A Primer of Water, Electrolyte and Acid-Base Syndromes, ed. 5. Lea and Febiger, Philadelphia, 1975.

Janz, G. J., and Tomkins, R. P. T.: Nonaqueous Electrolyte Handbook. Academic Press, New York, 1973.

Metheny, N. M., and Snively, W. D., Jr.: Nurses' Handbook of Fluid Balance, ed. 2. J. B. Lippincott Company, Philadelphia, 1974.

Scribner, B. H. and Burnell, J. M.: Teaching Syllabus for the Course on Fluid and Electrolyte Balance, ed. 7. University of Washington, Seattle, 1969.

NOTES

8

Calcium

Calcium is an important cation in relation to neuromuscular irritability, formation of bones and teeth, and the clotting of blood. The calcium level in the blood is controlled through the hormonal activity of the parathyroids. The parathyroids maintain a balance between calcium and phosphorus. Calcium should be ingested daily, since it is excreted daily in both the feces and the urine. Adequate vitamin D and protein are necessary for the utilization of calcium.

Distribution in the Body

The adult human body contains about 1200 grams of calcium, the majority (90%) being deposited in the bones as phosphate and carbonate. Very little calcium is present in the serum. However, when the serum level deviates from the normal range of 8.5 to 10.5 mg per cent, significant changes occur. About one half of serum calcium is free (ionized); the remainder is bound to plasma proteins, primarily albumin. It is *ionized* calcium that is measured by the serum calcium reading. When the serum calcium level falls, the bones and teeth are a ready source of calcium.

Functions

Calcium is important in the initiation of muscular contraction. When calcium enters the muscle fiber, it combines with special molecules to activate adenosine triphosphate (ATP), the energy source of all cells. The muscle stays contracted until the energy source is depleted or the calcium leaves the fluids as it is attracted away by the relaxing factor.

Calcium also interacts with the cell membranes of the nervous system so that the membranes are not overly charged.

Calcium performs an extremely important function in the coagulation of blood, since it participates in the reaction which converts prothrombin, a blood protein, into thrombin.

Calcium also strengthens the capillary membrane.

The most common function associated with calcium is, of course, its role in the formation of bones and teeth.

Calcium Excess

Excess calcium in the serum is called **hypercalcemia.** Calcium excesses are usually associated with metabolic changes such as those resulting from hyperparathyroidism, parathyroid tumor, or excessive administration of vitamin D. Calcium excess may also result from renal diseases in which the calcium cannot be properly excreted. Prolonged immobilization also encourages calcium retention. During immobilization, calcium moves from the bones, teeth, and intestines into the bloodstream. Calcium may also move to sites of malignant tumor formation, such as in the lungs, stomach, and kidneys.

Recognition. Significant signs and symptoms of calcium excess include neuromuscular changes, hypotonicity of the muscles, and deep bone and flank pain. Renal stones may occur because of the excretion of a high concentration of calcium through the parenchyma of the kidneys. **Polyuria** may be present, and some gastrointestinal symptoms may appear. These include anorexia, nausea, vomiting, thirst, and constipation. Constipation is related to the hypotonicity of muscles, when the smooth muscles of the gastrointestinal tract lack the necessary tension for adequate peristalsis. Bone cavitation may occur. The first sign of calcium imbalance may be the occurrence of a pathological fracture which can be related to the problems of a calcium excess. As the calcium level increases, the nervous system becomes depressed, producing lethargy, psychosis, and coma.

Laboratory Tests. The Sulkowitch urine test will reveal a high level of calcium in the urine. The serum calcium level will be above 10.5 mg per cent. An EKG can also be useful in diagnosing a calcium excess. Since the heart over-contracts when an excess of calcium is present, the EKG will indicate neuroelectrical changes in the heart.

Treatment. Treatment is directed toward the cause of the calcium excess. If immobilization can be corrected, the calcium excess will decrease. If a parathyroid tumor exists, its removal will correct the problem, although calcium replacement may be necessary after the surgery.

Treatment can include the administration of saline and sodium sulfate to cause diuresis and thereby encourage renal excretion of calcium. This treatment lessens the problem until the underlying cause can be diagnosed. Intravenous or oral phosphate may also be administered to induce calcium excretion. When the phosphorus level is elevated, calcium is released through the kidneys.

Steroids relieve the stress due to inflammation and thus tend to lessen the calcium mobilization which occurs in response to stress. Steroids also inhibit the absorption of calcium.

Since elevated calcium enhances digitalis intoxication, dosages of digitalis preparations may need to be decreased until the hypercalcemic state is improved.

In summary, treatment of calcium excess should be directed to the underlying causative condition. If other imbalances exist, the physician will give careful consideration to them before prescribing corrective treatments for the calcium excess.

Nurse's Responsibilities. Encourage mobility when possible.

Assist patient with passive exercises when mobility is impossible (if not in disagreement with the therapy regimen).

Strain urine to check for kidney stones.

Observe for symptoms implying the passage of a kidney stone.

Observe for central nervous and musculoskeletal system changes.

Calcium Deficit

A calcium deficit in the serum is called **hypocalcemia** and may be caused by a variety of problems.

Deficits can result from excessive gastrointestinal losses during diarrhea. Extraction of calcium from the extracellular fluid, such as occurs in acute pancreatitis or massive infections of the subcutaneous tissues, is another major cause of calcium loss. During pancreatic diseases, calcium is withdrawn from the extracellular fluid but is not absorbed by the intestines and is, therefore, lost with the feces. In a stress situation, the serum calcium level may decrease because calcium is mobilized from storage in the bones and teeth and is carried to the site of the injury or excreted. Excessive protein in the diet (protein greater than 0.9 to 1.0 mg/kg of body weight) will move calcium out of the bones allowing it to be excreted through the urine. Deficiency of bone calcium causes osteoporosis. The calcium level will also be decreased during the diuretic phase of renal failure. Since the parathyroids maintain an adequate calcium level in the blood, a deficit usually follows a thyroidectomy in which all four parathyroids have been removed.

Recognition. Symptoms of calcium deficit include muscle cramps, tetany, and convulsions due to changes in the neuromuscular irritability. Lack of calcium causes the membranes of nerve fibers to become partially charged; this results in the transmission of repetitive and uncontrolled impulses and leads to spasms of several muscle groups. A decreased calcium level causes the contraction of the heart muscle to be weak. Bleeding may be observed, and if the blood calcium level is extremely low, changes in clotting may be observed.

A calcium deficit may be suspected if the test for Trousseau's sign is positive. The carpopedal spasm (hand folding in) of Trousseau's sign may be observed while the arm is constricted with a blood pressure cuff.

Chvostek's sign can also indicate a calcium deficit. To obtain Chvostek's sign, tap the face over the facial nerve, which is in front of the temple; if the face twitches, the results are positive. Both of these signs are indicative of a serum calcium deficit. The diagnosis can be confirmed by testing the serum level. The normal serum calcium level is 8.5 to 10.5 mg per cent on the SMA 12.

Treatment. The treatment of hypocalcemia includes administration of calcium intravenously or orally. Vitamin D may need to be increased as well, since vitamin D aids in the absorption of calcium from the intestinal tract. In an acute calcium deficit, calcium should be given intravenously using a 10 per cent solution of calcium gluconate or gluceptate. This treatment is especially necessary if the patient has had tetany or a convulsion.

Nurse's Responsibilities. Observe for changes in neuromuscular irritability.

Place the patient on seizure precaution care.

Reduce stimuli as much as possible.

Administer digitalis preparations with caution.

Have a tracheotomy tray available.

BIBLIOGRAPHY

Bondy, P. K., and Rosenburg, L. E. (ed.): Duncan's Diseases of Metabolism, ed. 7. W. B. Saunders Company, Philadelphia, 1974.

Chakmakjian, Z. H., and Bethune, J. E.: Sodium sulfate treatment of hypercalcemia. N. Engl. J. Med. 275:862, 1966.

Goldberger, E.: A Primer of Water, Electrolyte and Acid-Base Syndromes, ed. 5. Lea and Febiger, Philadelphia, 1975.

Janz, G. J., and Tomkins, R. P. T.: Nonaqueous Electrolytes Handbook, ed. 2. Academic Press, New York, 1973.

Krupp, M. A., et al.: Physician's Handbook, ed. 17. Lange Medical Publications, Los Altos, California, 1973.

Metheny, N. M., and Snively, W. D., Jr.: Nurses' Handbook of Fluid Balance, ed. 2. J. B. Lippincott Company, Philadelphia, 1974.

Paton, R. R., Hegstrom, R. M., and Orme, B. M.: Fluid-Electrolyte Disorders. Mason Clinic, Seattle, 1969.

Rosenfeld, M. G. (ed.): Manual of Medical Therapeutics, ed. 20. Little,
Brown and Company, Boston, 1971.

Scribner, B. H., and Burnell, J. M.: Teaching Syllabus for the Course on
Fluid and Electrolyte Balance, ed. 7. University of Washington, Seattle, 1969.

Strott, C. A., and Nugent, C. A.: Laboratory test in diagnosis of hyperparathyroidism and hypercalcemic states. Ann. Intern. Med. 68:188,
1968.

NOTES

NOTES

SECTION IV

ACID-BASE

9

Acid-Base Balance

The ratio of acids and bases is closely related to the chemical balance in the body. This balance is extremely intricate and must be kept within the very slight margin of 7.35 to 7.45 pH in the extracellular fluid. The pH of the body is slightly alkaline. A chemically neutral solution is 7.00; 1.00 to 7.00 is acid; 7.00 to 14.00 is basic or alkaline.

Basic Concepts

Acids are **hydrogen ion** (proton) donors (see Fig. 9-1). This means that acids have hydrogen ions which will be given up to neutralize or decrease the strength of a base. For example, hydrochloric acid when mixed with sodium bicarbonate yields sodium chloride and carbonic acid. Hydrochloric acid donates its hydrogen proton to the sodium bicarbonate solution; this results in

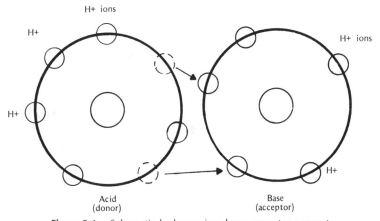

Figure 9-1. Schematic hydrogen ion donor-acceptor concept.

the neutralization of sodium bicarbonate to a salt, sodium chloride, and the formation of a weaker acid, carbonic acid.

Bases are proton or hydrogen ion acceptors (see Fig. 9-1). In the above example, the base, sodium bicarbonate, accepted the hydrogen proton from the hydrochloric acid thus converting the strong acid, hydrochloric acid, to the weaker acid, carbonic acid.

Note that the terms hydrogen-ion donor and acceptor are *not* synonymous with the terms cation and anion. Sodium and potassium are neither bases nor acids; the cation ammonium is a weak acid; the anions chloride and sulfate are weak bases; and at a blood pH level of 7.35 to 7.45, the anion bicarbonate is a weak base and the anion phosphoric acid is a weak acid. As you can see, there is no correlation between the positive or negative charge of an electrolyte and its capacity as a hydrogen ion donor or acceptor.

Regulatory Systems

The body controls the pH balance by the use of regulatory systems. These regulatory systems are the chemical **buffers,** the lungs, the cells, and the kidneys, in that order of control. The buffer systems are the fastest acting defenses, providing immediate protection against changes in the hydrogen ion concentration of the extracellular fluid. The buffers also serve as transport mechanisms that carry excess hydrogen ions to the lungs. The other regulatory systems are slower to react but provide more thorough protection.

A buffer is a substance that reacts to keep the pH within the narrow limits of stability when either too much acid or too much base is released into the system. Because a buffer is a reactor, it only functions when too much acid or base is present.

The chemicals in the buffer system are paired; a weakly ionized acid (or base) is balanced with a fully ionized salt. This combination is able to resist gross changes in the pH balance because when a strong acid (or base) is added, the weak acid (or base) already present is capable of neutralizing the additional hydrogen ions. In other words, the buffer acts as a chemical sponge absorbing or releasing hydrogen ions as needed.

There are three primary buffer systems in the extracellular fluid: the hemoglobin, the plasma protein, and the bicarbonate systems. These substances react immediately with acids or bases to minimize changes in the pH. However, once they react, they are consumed. This leaves the body less able to withstand a further stress until they are replaced.

1. Hemoglobin in the red blood cells helps maintain the acid-base balance by a process called chloride shift. Chloride shifts in and out of the red blood cells according to the level of oxygen in the blood plasma. For each chloride ion that leaves the red blood cell, a bicarbonate ion enters the cell, and vice-versa; i.e., for each chloride ion which enters the red blood cell, a bicarbonate ion is released.

2. Plasma protein functions in conjunction with the liver to vary the amount of hydrogen ions in the chemical structure of the protein. Plasma protein has the ability to attract or release hydrogen ions.

3. The bicarbonate buffer system maintains the blood pH at 7.4 with a ratio of twenty parts bicarbonate to one part carbonic acid. (see Fig. 9-2). If a strong acid is added to the body, the ratio is upset because some of the bicarbonate will be lost in the process of neutralizing the strong acid to the weaker one, carbonic acid.

The regulatory systems of the body interact to maintain the pH balance. The lungs, which are the body's next defense in acid-base balance after the chemical buffers, interact with the buffer system to perform their function. The carbonic acid which, as just mentioned, was created by the neutralizing action of the bicarbonate, can be carried to the lungs where it is reduced to carbon dioxide and water, both of which are exhaled. In this way, the hydrogen ions are inactivated and excreted.

When there is a bicarbonate excess, the lungs, which have the ability to

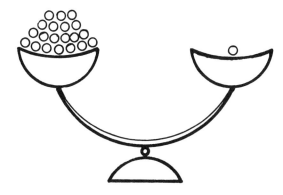

20 bicarbonates : 1 carbonic acid

Figure 9-2. Acid-base balance. Blood pH is 7.4.

regulate the speed and depth of respirations, suppress respiration to allow a build-up of carbonic acid. The carbonic acid then serves to neutralize and decrease the strength of the excess bicarbonate. The action of the lungs is reversible, making it possible for them to control an excess or deficit. This means that the lungs can either hold the hydrogen ions until the deficit is corrected, or they can inactivate the hydrogen ions into water molecules to be exhaled with the carbon dioxide as vapor, thereby correcting the excess. It takes from 10 to 30 minutes for the lungs to inactivate the hydrogen molecules by converting them to water molecules. The lungs are capable of inactivating only those hydrogen ions carried by carbonic acid. Excess hydrogen ions created by other problems must be excreted through the kidneys.

The cells can also serve as regulators or buffers. They react in two to four hours, and they have the ability to soak up or release extra hydrogen ions. Potassium plays an exchange role in maintaining the correct hydrogen ion level (see Chapter 5).

The ultimate correction of acid-base disturbances and the restoration of buffers are dependent upon the kidneys, even though renal excretion of acids and, to a lesser degree, alkali occurs more slowly. Compensation through the kidneys requires a period of a few hours to several days. However, renal action is more thorough and selective than that of other acid-base regulators. The primary mechanism of the kidneys in acid-base balance is the selective regulation of bicarbonate. The kidneys restore bicarbonate by releasing hydrogen ions and holding bicarbonate ions. The secondary and tertiary mechanisms involve the acids secreted by the renal tubular cells. In the second mechanism, the buffer, primarily phosphate, becomes acidic, and the extra hydrogen ions are excreted in the urine in the form of phosphoric acid. The third mechanism, which also involves a chemical change within the renal tubules, is called the ammonia mechanism. The alteration of certain amino acids in the renal tubules results in a diffusion of ammonia into the kidneys where it picks up excess hydrogen ions and is excreted as ammonium. Both phosphoric acid and ammonium are fixed acids.

Because fixed acids cannot be destroyed in metabolism nor eliminated through the lungs, they must instead be excreted through the kidneys. Thus the kidneys are very important in the regulation of pH balance. The urine can sustain a hydrogen concentration a thousand times greater than can the blood. The maximum urine acidity is pH 4.0 compared to the normal blood pH of 7.4. However, very little acid can be excreted by the kidneys as free hydrogen ions but instead must be excreted as fixed acids and ammonium in approximately equal amounts.

BIBLIOGRAPHY

Bland, J. H.: Clinical Metabolism of Water and Electrolytes. W. B. Saunders Company, Philadelphia, 1963.

Blumenthals, A. S.: Symposium on acid base balance. Arch. Intern. Med. 116:647, 1965.

Bondy, P. K., and Rosenburg, L. E. (eds.): Duncan's Diseases of Metabolism, ed. 7. W. B. Saunders Company, Philadelphia, 1974.

Davenport, H. W.: ABC of Acid-Base Chemistry: The Elements of Physiological Blood-Gas Chemistry for Medical Students and Physicians, ed. 6. University of Chicago Press, Chicago, 1974.

Frisell, W. R.: Acid-Base Chemistry in Medicine. The Macmillan Company, New York, 1968.

Goldberger, E.: A Primer of Water, Electrolyte, and Acid-Base Syndromes, ed. 5. Lea and Febiger, Philadelphia, 1975.

Guyton, A. C.: Function of the Human Body, ed. 4. W. B. Saunders Company, Philadelphia, 1974.

Kee, J. L.: Fluids and Electrolytes with Clinical Applications: A Programmed Approach. John Wiley and Sons, Inc., New York, 1971.

Maxwell, M. H., and Kleeman, C. R.: Clinical Disorders of Fluid and Electrolyte Metabolism, ed. 2. McGraw-Hill Book Company, New York, 1972.

Metheny, N. M., and Snively, W. D., Jr.: Nurses' Handbook of Fluid Balance, ed. 2. J. B. Lippincott Company, Philadelphia, 1974.

Paton, R. R., Hegstrom, R. M., and Orme, B. M.: Fluid-Electrolyte Disorders. Mason Clinic, Seattle, 1969.

Pitts, R. F.: Physiology of the Kidney and Body Fluids, ed. 3. Year Book Medical Publishers, Inc., Chicago, 1974.

Ravel, R.: Clinical Laboratory Medicine. Year Book Medical Publishers, Chicago, 1972.

Rosenfeld, M. G. (ed.): Manual of Medical Therapeutics, ed. 20. Little, Brown and Company, Boston, 1971.

Scribner, B. H., and Burnell, J. M.: Teaching Syllabus for the Course on Fluid and Electrolyte Balance, ed. 7. University of Washington, Seattle, 1969.

Takacs, F. J.: Metabolic alkalosis. Hosp. Med. 4:61, 1968.

Wesson, L. G.: Physiology of the Human Kidney. Grune and Stratton, Inc., New York, 1969.

NOTES

88

NOTES

10

Metabolic Acidosis and Alkalosis

We have established that the normal blood pH is maintained between 7.35 and 7.45 by the regulatory systems. When the pH drops below 7.35, this condition is referred to as acidosis. Thus acidosis is a condition in which the total concentration of the **buffer base** is reduced below normal, leaving a relatively higher concentration of hydrogen ions. As a result, a greater number of hydrogen ions are circulating in the blood than can be absorbed by the buffering systems. The signs and symptoms show how the body further attempts to cope with or compensate for this increase in hydrogen concentration by further activating the lungs, the cells, and the kidneys.

Alkalosis is the condition in which the pH is above 7.45. In this condition, the total concentration of buffer base is greater than normal with a relative decrease in the hydrogen ion concentration. Thus in alkalosis too much base exists while the acid concentration is reduced.

There are two major types of acidosis and alkalosis: respiratory and metabolic. Respiratory acid-base imbalances are caused by primary defects in the function of the lungs or changes in the normal respiratory patterns due to secondary problems. Respiratory acidosis and alkalosis are discussed in Chapter 11.

Metabolic acidosis and alkalosis are due primarily to changes in the burning and utilization of particular nutrients. Metabolic acid-base imbalances are the subject of this chapter.

METABOLIC ACIDOSIS

Metabolic acidosis is a primary base deficit or an accumulation of fixed **(nonvolatile)** acids. In other words, acidosis may be a result of losing too many bases or of holding too many acids (see Fig. 10-1). Without sufficient bases, the pH of the blood will be acidotic, i.e., below 7.35.

Causes

Table 10-1 outlines causes of metabolic acidosis.

Recognition

Signs and symptoms indicative of metabolic acidosis include headache, drowsiness, nausea, vomiting, diarrhea, stupor, coma, twitching, and convulsions. Acidosis that results from improper fat metabolism often produces a

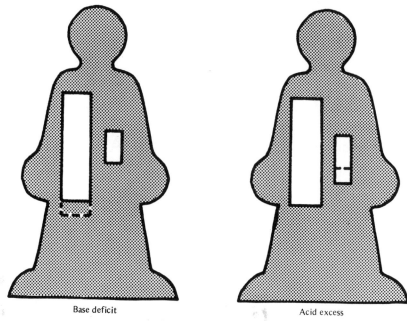

Base deficit   Acid excess

Figure 10-1. Acidosis.

TABLE 10-1. CAUSES OF METABOLIC ACIDOSIS

Cause	Altered Function
Diabetes (diabetic ketoacidosis)	Insufficient insulin results in increased fat metabolism which produces excess accumulation of ketones, acetoacetic acids, acetone, and other acids.
Renal insufficiency/failure (renal acidosis)	Increased waste products of protein metabolism (urea, creatinine, phosphoric acid, sulfuric acid) are retained; excessive acids decrease the bicarbonate available to maintain acid-base balance.
Incomplete metabolism of carbohydrates (lactic acidosis)	Insufficient oxygen for proper burning of carbohydrates to glucose and water; therefore lactic acid increases
Salicylate intoxication	Excessive ingestion of acetylsalicylic acid
Severe diarrhea	Intestinal and pancreatic secretions are normally alkaline, therefore excessive base loss results in acidosis.
Malnutrition	Improper metabolism of nutrients; fat catabolism results in excess ketones and acids
High fat diet	Too rapid accumulation of the waste products of fat metabolism (ketones)
Addison's disease (terminal)	Insufficient amount of sodium and chloride held by the body with build up of potassium due to lack of adrenocortical steroids (glucocorticoids and mineralcorticoids)

fruity smelling breath in the patient. Hyperpnea may also be present, indicating an attempt by the body to ''blow off'' extra carbon dioxide which, if retained, forms an acid in the serum. This type of respiration is usually known as Kussmaul's respiration.

Laboratory Tests

The pH level will be below 7.35, indicating that there are either more hydrogen ions or less bicarbonate ions present in the blood. The serum carbon dioxide (CO_2) level will be decreased below 22 mEq/L. It is not unusual for this reading to be proportionately more reduced in metabolic acidosis than in respiratory acidosis. The serum carbon dioxide (CO_2) reading primarily measures the amount of circulating bicarbonate. Since this is one of the main buffers, the reading will be decreased because bicarbonate has been depleted in the neutralization of the extra acid. The partial pressure of the blood gas carbon dioxide **(pCO_2)** will decrease below 35 to 40 millimeters of pressure if the patient is compensating for the acidosis by increasing the respiratory rate. This is an important concept in understanding the compensatory function of the lungs. In metabolic acidosis, the lungs increase their rate in order to ''blow off'' acids, thereby reducing acidosis. (In contrast, during respiratory acidosis, the kidneys perform the **compensation.**) The partial pressure of oxygen **(pO_2)** is usually increased due to hyperpnea. The normal partial pressure of oxygen is 90 to 100 millimeters of pressure. Sodium and chloride levels may be decreased, while the serum potassium level is increased with acidosis.

Treatment

In most cases, acidosis will be treated according to the underlying cause. However, there are some guidelines to follow regarding acidosis in general. An emergency alkalinization of a patient can be accomplished quickly by administering a bicarbonate solution, usually intravenously, to add to the buffer base of the blood. The solution usually given is sodium bicarbonate, 1 to 3 ampules (50 mEq $NaHCO_3$/ampule).

The potassium level in the serum should be closely monitored when acidosis is being treated, since potassium will move back into the cell and may become too low. This is especially true if potassium has been lost through the urine and gastrointestinal tract.

An intravenous solution, such as isotonic saline, 5 per cent dextrose in 0.45 per cent saline, sodium lactate, or bicarbonate may be used to increase the base level. Lactate and bicarbonate are the primary treatments. The liver converts sodium lactate to bicarbonate.

Insulin administered for diabetes mellitus will hasten the movement of glucose out of the serum and into the cell, thereby lessening any concurrent ketosis. When glucose is being properly metabolized, the body will stop converting the fats to glucose. Insulin lessens ketones by decreasing the release of fatty acids from fat cells. In diabetes, it is also necessary to watch for circulatory collapse due to the polyuria which may result from the hyperglycemic state. Polyuria or diuresis may lead to an extracellular volume deficit. In attempting to correct the hyperglycemic state, Levophed or **catecholamines** administered to correct the hypovolemia must be used carefully, because these treatments may cause lactic acidosis in the diabetic.

In renal failure, dialysis can be used to remove the protein waste products and thereby lessen the acidotic state. A diet low in protein and high in calories (carbohydrates and fats) will lessen the amount of protein waste products due to protein catabolism. This, in turn, will help lessen the acidosis. Although the prognosis is poor for the patient with lactic acidosis, the administration of oxygen will help to adjust the lactic acidotic state.

In Addison's disease, treatment consists of replacing the steroids.

Nurse's Responsibilities

Have sodium bicarbonate ready for emergency administration.

Take safety precautions for convulsion or coma.

Maintain intake-output record to assist the physician in planning fluid replacement.

Observe skin, vital signs, and eye balls (sunken or protruding) as indicative of positive or negative changes in the patient.

METABOLIC ALKALOSIS

Metabolic alkalosis may result from one of two imbalances: a malfunction of metabolism, causing an increase in the amount of available basic solutions in the blood, or a reduction of available acids in the serum (see Fig. 10-2). Both of these abnormalities result in an increase in the blood pH to a level above 7.45.

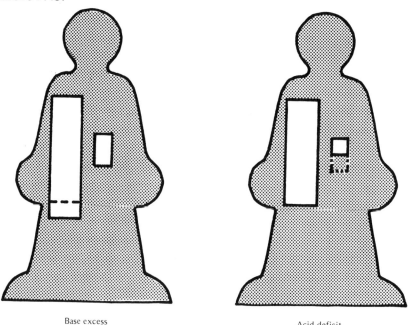

Base excess   Acid deficit

Figure 10-2. Alkalosis.

Causes

Table 10-2 outlines causes of metabolic alkalosis.

Laboratory Tests

The pH level will be above 7.45.

The serum carbon dioxide (CO_2) level will increase above 32 mEq/L because this test reflects the amount of circulating plasma bicarbonate (base). Properly functioning kidneys have the ability to secrete some of the bicarbonate.

TABLE 10-2. CAUSES OF METABOLIC ALKALOSIS

Cause	Altered Function
Ingestion of excess sodium bicarbonate	Rapid absorption of bicarbonate through gastric mucosa
Excessive vomiting	Loss of potassium and hydrochloric acid from the stomach
Gastrointestinal intubation (especially Levin tube) or gastric lavage	Loss of upper gastrointestinal secretions which are high in hydrochloric acid and secondarily in potassium
Administration of potent diuretics	Loss of hydrogen and chloride ions causes a compensatory increase of bicarbonate in the blood
Prolonged hypercalcemia	Relationship unidentified

The partial pressure of carbon dioxide (pCO_2) will not change unless the lungs attempt to compensate for the alkalosis. In *compensated* metabolic alkalosis, the partial pressure of carbon dioxide (pCO_2) will rise in an attempt to increase carbonic acid to a level where it will neutralize the basic state.

Serum potassium and chloride levels will be decreased. Note that the serum chloride reading will decrease *disproportionately* to a decreased serum sodium reading. In other imbalances, the sodium and chloride decrease in a proportionate ratio.

Recognition

The signs and symptoms of metabolic alkalosis are difficult to separate from other conditions occurring with the alkalosis, particularly the changes caused by potassium and chloride deficits. However, some of the major signs and symptoms the nurse should know are nausea, vomiting, and diarrhea. Such psychological symptoms as confusion, irritability, agitation leading to coma, and possible convulsions are not uncommon. In some cases, symptoms similar to those which accompany calcium imbalance may be present. These include restlessness and twitching of the extremities.

The EKG readings may show a sinus tachycardia. Another change in the EKG indicative of metabolic alkalosis is the low T wave merging with the P wave.

Treatment

The major impetus in the treatment of alkalosis is to correct the pH imbalance and eliminate the underlying cause of the alkalosis. However, prevention of alkalosis is even more urgent and, in many ways, easier to accomplish, as can be seen by reviewing the list of its causes. Someone taking soda for an ulcer or to alleviate an "acid stomach" should be reminded of the negative side effects of excessive ingestion of sodium bicarbonate and cautioned against consuming large amounts. If a patient with congestive heart failure is taking diuretic preparation, his potassium level should be checked frequently in order to alert the physician to a developing potassium deficit.

If preventive measures fail and corrective treatment should be initiated, there are several common alternate methods available. The method decided upon will depend upon the specific case.

Excessive losses of potassium and chloride should be replaced. This can be accomplished intravenously or orally, using foods such as fruits and meats which are high in potassium. Potassium replacement should be governed by the amounts of potassium and chloride lost in the secretions. Replacement needed can be calculated by two methods. Loss can be estimated according to a standard number of milliequivalents of electrolyte per liter of fluid. For example, the average amount of potassium per liter of gastric fluid loss is 5 to 10 mEq. The second method, whereby the exact milliequivalents per liter of fluid loss are measured in the laboratory, is more accurate.

Diamox may be given to promote kidney excretion of bicarbonate.

Acidifying solutions such as ammonium chloride and arginine chloride may be used intravenously or orally. The added hydrogen ions present in these solutions increase the available acids in the serum. Ammonium chloride is particularly helpful in an alkalosis caused by diuretics of the potent thiazide and mercurial groups.

Sodium chloride may be administered orally or intravenously, unless other conditions, such as congestive heart failure, are contraindicative.

Nurse's Responsibilities

Maintain accurate intake-output records, particularly to determine the electrolyte losses contributing to alkalosis; potassium and hydrogen ion losses are especially important.

Check for vital sign changes suggestive of hypokalemia.

Check for muscle weakness which may be related to hypokalemia.

Take safety precautions for the confusion often present in alkalotic patients.

Take seizure precautions for possible tetany and convulsions.

CASE STUDY 10.1

A 52-year-old woman was admitted to the hospital in a semicomatose condition. Her husband reported she had had the "flu" for four days prior to admission and had been vomiting. In spite of vomiting, she had continued to drink large quantities of water. She was a known diabetic.

Her pulse was weak and rapid, respirations were of the Kussmaul type, and blood pressure was normal.

Physician orders included 80 units of regular insulin stat, IV fluids with regular insulin, hourly urine tests for sugar and acetone with sliding scale of insulin.

Laboratory report: Blood sugar 454 mg %; CO_2 11 mEq/L; Na 130 mEq/L; Cl 93 mEq/L; K 7.6 mEq/L.
Blood gases: pH 7.27; pCO_2 24 mmHg; HCO_3 13.5 mEq/L; pO_2 91 mmHg.

Within 10 hours of admission, urinary output was 2350 cc.

Discussion Questions

1. When a patient is vomiting, how does continuing to drink large quantities of water affect the serum electrolyte values?

---

*For answers to Case Study Questions, see Appendix 4.

2. What effect does a high amount of blood sugar have on urinary output?

3. Evaluate the laboratory reports.

4. Describe the results of the low serum CO_2 in this particular case.

5. What treatment would correct this ketoacidosis?

Quiz 10.1*

A 52-year-old woman was admitted to the hospital in a semicomatose condition. Her husband reported she had had the "flu" and had been vomiting for four days. She had been drinking large quantities of water. She was a known diabetic.

Laboratory report: Blood sugar 454 mg %; CO_2 11 mEq/L; Na 130 mEq/L; Cl 93 mEq/L; K 7.6 mEq/L; pH 7.27; pCO_2 24 mmHg; HCO_3 13.5 mEq/L; PO_2 91 mmHg.

Check the following as true or false:

True	False		
_____	_____	1.	Glucose exerts a diuretic effect.
_____	_____	2.	Ketone bodies (acetone) result from incomplete fat metabolism.
_____	_____	3.	Ketosis induces vomiting.
_____	_____	4.	The low serum CO_2 indicates the patient has too little bicarbonate.
_____	_____	5.	The elevated potassium is due to the acidosis.
_____	_____	6.	This patient needed IV fluids with insulin stat.
_____	_____	7.	Insulin stops production of ketone bodies.
_____	_____	8.	Laboratories never make errors on electrolyte reports.

CASE STUDY 10.2

A 50-year-old man was admitted to the hospital with a hernia. He admitted to frequent laxative use and occasional diarrhea. Postoperatively he de-

*For answers to Quizzes, see Appendix 5.

veloped a **paralytic ileus;** a Levin tube was inserted to control vomiting. He was returned to surgery for an intestinal obstruction. Physician orders:
1000 cc Ringer's lactate with 40 mEq KCl every 8 hours.
Irrigate Levin tube.
May have ice chips.
Serum electrolyte report:
Na 130 mEq/L; K 3.0 mEq/L; Cl mEq/L; CO_2 44 mEq/L.

Questions

1. With the above information, what fluid and/or electrolyte or acid-base imbalances would you suspect?   Explain.

2. List abnormal electrolytes. What do they indicate?

The alert nurse should immediately slow the Ringer's lactate administration. A serum CO_2 level of 44 indicates an excess of bicarbonate. The lactate in the IV fluid would convert into bicarbonate in the liver causing a further deterioration of the patient's condition.

3. What kind and amount of solution should be used for Levin irrigation?   Why?

4. Discuss this patient's acid-base problem.

Quiz 10.2

A 50-year-old man was admitted to the hospital with a hernia. He admitted to frequent laxative use and occasional diarrhea. Postoperatively he developed a paralytic ileus, and a Levin tube was inserted to control vomiting. He was returned to surgery for an intestinal obstruction. Serum electrolyte report: Na 130 mEq/L; K 3.0 mEq/L; Cl 62 mEq/L; CO_2 44 mEq/L.

1. Evaluate:

	Normal	Increased	Decreased
ECF	_____	_____	_____
Na	_____	_____	_____
K	_____	_____	_____
Cl	_____	_____	_____
CO_2	_____	_____	_____

2. a. Levin tubes should be irrigated with:
      1. _____ normal saline
      2. _____ tap water
      3. _____ not irrigated
   b. Patients with Levin tubes should have:
      1. _____ no limit on their intake of water and ice chips.
      2. _____ minimal amounts of water and ice chips because liquids promote excessive intestinal secretion and loss of electrolytes.

3. In metabolic alkalosis the primary alteration is:
   a. _____ deficit of bicarbonate.
   b. _____ excess of bicarbonate.
   c. _____ deficit of carbonic acid.
   d. _____ excess of carbonic acid.

4. Which of the following laboratory reports show a metabolic alkalosis?
   a. _____ pH 7.16 pCO_2 58 pO_2 40 HCO_3 38
   b. _____ pH 7.50 pCO_2 25 pO_2 86 HCO_3 24
   c. _____ pH 7.16 pCO_2 25 pO_2 86 HCO_3 9
   d. _____ pH 7.50 pCO_2 45 pO_2 86 HCO_3 38

BIBLIOGRAPHY

Bland, J. H.: Clinical Metabolism of Water and Electrolytes. W. B. Saunders Company, Philadelphia, 1963.

Blumentals, A. S.: Symposium on acid base balance. Arch. Intern. Med. 116:647, 1965.

Davenport, H. W.: ABC of Acid-Base Chemistry: The Elements of Physiological Blood-Gas Chemistry for Medical Students and Physicians, ed. 6. University of Chicago Press, Chicago, 1974.

Frisell, W. R.: Acid-Base Chemistry in Medicine. The Macmillan Company, New York, 1968.

Goldberger, E.: A Primer of Water, Electrolyte, and Acid-Base Syndromes, ed. 5. Lea and Febiger, Philadelphia, 1975.

Maxwell, M. H., and Kleeman, C. R.: Clinical Disorders of Fluid & Electrolyte Metabolism, ed. 2. McGraw-Hill Book Company, New York, 1972.

Metheny, N. M., and Snively, W. D., Jr.: Nurses' Handbook of Fluid Balance, ed. 2. J. B. Lippincott Company, Philadelphia, 1974.

Paton, R. R., Hegstrom, R. M., and Orme, B. M.: Fluid-Electrolyte Disorders. Mason Clinic, Seattle, 1969.

Rosenfeld, M. G. (ed.): Manual of Medical Therapeutics, ed. 20. Little, Brown and Company, Boston, 1971.

Scribner, B. H., and Burnell, J. M.: Teaching Syllabus for the Course on Fluid and Electrolyte Balance, ed. 7. University of Washington, Seattle, 1969.

Takacs, Frank J.: Metabolic Alkalosis. Hosp. Med. 4:61, 1968.

NOTES

11

Respiratory Acidosis and Alkalosis

Respiratory acidosis and alkalosis, like metabolic acidosis and alkalosis, are the results of imbalances in the pH. Acidosis is a condition in which the total concentration of buffer base is below normal, with a relative increase in hydrogen ion concentration. Thus, a greater number of hydrogen ions are circulating in the blood than can be absorbed by the buffering systems. Alkalosis is a condition in which the total concentration of buffer base is greater than normal, with a relative decrease in hydrogen ion concentration. Thus in alkalosis there is too much base and too little acid concentration.

Respiratory imbalances are caused by primary defects in the function of the lungs or by changes in the normal respiratory pattern due to secondary problems. In either case, the result of the dysfunction is an increase or decrease in the serum concentration of carbonic acid (H_2CO_3).

RESPIRATORY ACIDOSIS

Carbon dioxide is a waste product that must be removed from the body. The lungs normally remove 15,000 to 20,000 mEq of hydrogen ions per day as carbon dioxide gas. Respiratory acidosis is caused when carbon dioxide, which is a volatile substance, is retained due to hypoventilation (see Fig. 11-1).

The suppression of respiration causes retention of carbon dioxide which combines with water to form carbonic acid. This increased acid causes the pH reading to decrease, creating the acidotic state.

Causes

Table 11-1 lists the causes and altered functions of respiratory acidosis.

Recognition

Signs and symptoms indicating respiratory acidosis include decreased ventilation, somnolence, and sensorium changes. As hypoxia becomes more acute, such recognizable conditions as diaphoresis, cyanosis, restlessness, and rapid, irregular pulse may occur. The rapid pulse may lead to an arrhythmia. Cyanosis is a *late* sign.

Laboratory Tests

The pH will be below 7.35, indicating that the concentration of carbonic

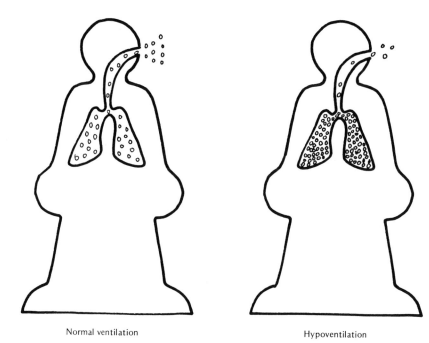

Normal ventilation   Hypoventilation

Figure 11-1.   Hypoventilation.

acid in the serum is increased. The blood gas carbon dioxide (pCO_2) will be over 40 mmHg. The partial pressure of oxygen (pO_2) will be normal (90 to 100) or decreased (90 to 60) as the hypoxia increases. A pO_2 60 mmHg or below must be reported because of possible arrhythmias. The bicarbonate level will be normal if the respiratory acidosis is uncompensated; it will be elevated with partial or complete compensation. The kidneys can compensate for respiratory acidosis; however, it takes from a few hours to several days for compensation to take place. To compensate for respiratory acidosis, the kidneys retain bicarbonate and return it to the extracellular fluid compartment. Usually conditions of chronic obstructive pulmonary disease (COPD) will show a partial compensation with a serum bicarbonate reading above 30 mEq/L. This elevated reading reflects the action of the kidneys which are retaining bicarbonate to buffer or neutralize the excess acids. Serum potassium will be elevated, relative to the potassium level before the acidosis developed.

Treatment

Since respiratory acidosis can develop very quickly into an emergency situation, the goal of primary importance is to improve ventilation and increase aeration by whatever means the clinical picture suggests. Intermittent positive pressure breathing (IPPB), antibiotics, and postural drainage are commonly used, followed by the insertion of an endotracheal tube, tracheotomy, and/or assisted or controlled ventilation when necessary.

Tranquilizers, narcotics, and hypnotics will further depress respiration and should be avoided.

Nurse's Responsibilities

Encourage and assist the patient to turn, cough, and breathe deeply frequently.

TABLE 11-1. CAUSES OF RESPIRATORY ACIDOSIS

Cause	Altered Function
Chronic diseases	
Emphysema	Loss of elasticity in alveolar sacs; destruction dominant over obstruction; restricted air flow in and out, primarily out, results in elevated pCO_2
Asthma	Spasms due to allergens, irritants, or emotions cause smooth muscles of bronchioles to constrict
Bronchitis	Inflammation obstructs airway
Pulmonary edema	ECF accumulation in acute congestive heart failure causes decreased alveolar diffusion and perfusion
Bronchiectasis	Bronchi dilated due to inflammation; destructive changes and weakness in walls of bronchi
Acute diseases	
Infection	Aeration decreased due to obstruction of airway caused by inflammation and bacterial agents
Sedatives (narcotics)	Depressed respiratory center leads to CO_2 narcosis
Pneumonia	Inadequate oxygenation due to fluid accumulation caused by infection, irritants, immobility
Atelectasis	Excessive mucus with collapse of alveolar sacs due to mucus plugs, infectious drainage or anesthetic drugs causes decreased respiration
Brain trauma	Excessive pressure on respiratory center, medulla oblongata, depresses respiration

Use suction as necessary.

Encourage proper hydration to thin secretions unless contraindicated.

Reduce restlesness by improving ventilation rather than by administering narcotics and sedatives.

Maintain oxygen flow as ordered.

Report signs of respiratory distress promptly.

Be alert to increased pulse rate.

Perform chest physiotherapy (cupping and clapping) and postural drainage as ordered.

Place in semi-Fowler's position unless contraindicated.

RESPIRATORY ALKALOSIS

Respiratory alkalosis is due to hyperventilation. Rapid respiration causes expiration of an increased amount of carbon dioxide, resulting in a deficit of carbonic acid (Fig. 11-2). It is often **neurogenic** in origin.

Figure 11-2. Hyperventilation.

Causes

Table 11-2 lists causes and altered functions of respiratory alkalosis.

TABLE 11-2. CAUSES OF RESPIRATORY ALKALOSIS

Cause	*Altered Function*
Hysteria	Psychoneurosis causes vigorous breathing resulting in excessive exhaling of CO_2 (hyperventilation)
Pain; brain trauma	Overstimulation of respiratory center with resultant H_2CO_3 deficit (hyperventilation)
Drugs (acetylsalicylic acid)	Salicylates initially stimulate respiratory center causing hyperventilation; secondary development of metabolic acidosis with compensatory hyperventilation
Oxygen-lack	Hypoxia may cause respiratory stimulation with resultant H_2CO_3 deficit (hyperventilation)
Ventilators	Iatrogenic; overadministration of O_2 and depletion of pCO_2 occurs while adjusting ventilator to the patient (hyperventilation)

Recognition

Respiratory alkalosis can be recognized by the abnormally rapid respiration that accompanies hyperventilation. The causes listed in Table 11-2 may precede or accompany hyperventilation. The patient may experience headache, vertigo, paresthesias, tetany, carpopedal spasms, and **syncope.**

Laboratory
Tests

The pH will be above 7.45, indicating a decreased concentration of carbonic acid in the serum. The blood gas carbon dioxide (pCO_2), will be below 40 mmHg. The partial pressure of oxygen will probably be normal. The bicarbonate level will be normal if the respiratory alkalosis is uncompensated; it will be lowered with compensation. The kidneys compensate for respiratory alkalosis by decreasing both tubular acid secretion and reabsorption of bicarbonate. In other words, the kidneys retain hydrogen ions and excrete bicarbonate in proportion to the amount of carbon dioxide that has been ''blown off'' during hyperventilation. The serum potassium level will be lowered, and the urine will be alkaline.

Treatment

The common treatment is sedation and reassurance, CO_2 treatments, voluntary breath-holding, or use of a rebreathing mask.

Nurse's Responsibilities

Provide emotional support and educate patient regarding breathing patterns.
Administer medications as ordered.
Be alert to signs and symptoms of other disease processes that could be masked by the more obvious symptoms of respiratory alkalosis.
Encourage breathing techniques and apply breathing aids as indicated.

CASE STUDY 11.1*

A 54-year-old man was admitted to the hospital with acute bronchitis. The admission orders included Thorazine 50 mg IM stat, IPPB with Isuprel tid for 10 minutes, Carbrital FS cap.I at HS and may repeat X 1. Additional orders later in the day included O_2 5 L/min per nasal cannula, Thorazine 25 mg orally tid, Aminophyllin 10 cc IV for extreme respiratory distress, Demerol 100 mg IM q 6 hours prn pain, and ASA gr X prn for temperature over 101°. Vital signs: BP 152/108; P 124; R 24; T 98.4.

Questions

1. List nursing responsibilities upon admission of this patient.

2. Should the nurse question the physician's order for oxygen at 5 L/min?

3. What can the nurse do to improve aeration?

---
*For answers to Case Study Questions, see Appendix 4.

4. Early the next morning, the patient developed sensorium changes (confusion), diaphoresis, increased congestion, and then ceased to respond. He was given Aminophyllin 10 cc IV. Stat electrolytes and blood gas test reports were as follows:
Na 143 mEq/L; K 5.3 mEq/L; Cl 104 mEq/L; CO_2 44 mEq/L; BUN 16 mg %; pH 7.27; pCO_2 72 mmHg; pO_2 108 mmHg.
a) Why was Aminophyllin given?

b) Evaluate the electrolyte and blood gas reports.

5. Why did the physician discontinue the Thorazine, Carbrital, ASA, and Demerol, and leave a new order for no sedatives?

6. It has been stated in previous chapters that potassium becomes elevated in acidosis. Explain this patient's normal potassium with the severe respiratory acidosis.

7. The patient appeared less alert following IPPB treatments and upon questioning stated that he blacked out during these treatments. Explain.

Quiz 11.1*

A 54-year-old man was admitted to the hospital with a diagnosis of COPD (chronic obstructive pulmonary disease) and acute bronchitis. Laboratory reports: Na 143 mEq/L; K 5.3 mEq/L; Cl 104 mEq/L; CO_2 44 mEq/L; BUN 16 mg %; pH 7.27; pCO_2 72 mmHg; pO_2 108 mmHg.

Check the following true or false:

True	False	
_____	_____	1. Acute respiratory diseases show signs of decreased aeration; a high flow of O_2 will correct this.

_____   _____   2. This patient developed an increased concentration of carbonic acid (H_2CO_3) in his serum.

_____   _____   3. Aminophyllin is compatible with adrenalin.

_____   _____   4. Patients with COPD usually show a renal compensation by an increased serum CO_2 level.

_____   _____   5. Sedation will relax this patient, and he will breathe easier.

_____   _____   6. Acute respiratory failure is life-threatening.

_____   _____   7. The function of ventilation is to maintain a high CO_2 and a low O_2.

Correlate the disease with the ventilation problem:

8. _____ bronchial asthma   a. airway obstruction

9. _____ acute bronchitis   b. diffusion defect

10. _____ emphysema   c. perfusion problem

11. _____ acute pulmonary edema

12. _____ pulmonary embolism

**CASE STUDY
11.2**

A 48-year-old man was admitted to the hospital complaining of abdominal pain. He appeared apprehensive. Other complaints were abdominal bloating and back pain. Shortness of breath was determined to be "functional" by the physician. Stat laboratory test reports were as follows: pH 7.58; pCO_2 22 mmHg; pO_2 77 mmHg; BUN 64 mg %; creatinine 2.5 mg %.

Questions

1. Analyze the laboratory report.

2. What is hyperventilation?

3. Are hypoxia and ventilation synonymous?

4. What is the most common treatment for respiratory alkalosis caused by anxiety or hysteria?

5. Discuss mechanical ventilators in relation to respiratory alkalosis.

Several days after admission this patient suffered a cardiac arrest; it was determined that he had had an unrecognized acute myocardial infarction. The respiratory alkalosis apparently masked his other symptoms which were nonclassical for a myocardial infarction.

Quiz 11.2

A 48-year-old man was admitted to the hospital complaining of abdominal pain, abdominal bloating, back pain, and shortness of breath. He appeared apprehensive. The physician determined the symptoms to be "functional." Laboratory test reports were: pH 7.58; pCO_2 22 mmHg; pO_2 77 mmHg; BUN 64 mg %; creatinine 2.5 mg %.

1. A pH over 7.5 is called _____.
2. True   False

   _____   _____   a. Respiratory alkalosis is always an emergency situation.
   _____   _____   b. The kidneys compensate in respiratory acidosis/alkalosis.
   _____   _____   c. CO_2 by mask and breathing into a paper bag are common treatments for functional respiratory alkalosis.
   _____   _____   d. Carbon dioxide dilates peripheral blood vessels.

3. Match the diagnosis with the proper laboratory results:

   __e__ Respiratory acidosis   a. pH 7.52 pCO_2 45 pO_2 88 HCO_3 36
   __b__ Metabolic acidosis   b. pH 7.15 pCO_2 24 pO_2 88 HCO_3 8
   __D__ Respiratory alkalosis   c. pH 7.42 pCO_2 40 pO_2 88 HCO_3 25
   __A__ Metabolic alkalosis   d. pH 7.52 pCO_2 24 pO_2 88 HCO_3 22
                                 e. pH 7.15 pCO_2 60 pO_2 40 HCO_3 39

BIBLIOGRAPHY

Bates, D. V., Macklem, P. T., and Christie, R. V.: Respiratory Function in Disease: An Introduction to the Integrated Study of the Lung, ed. 2. W. B. Saunders Company, Philadelphia, 1971.

Chronic Obstructive Pulmonary Disease, ed. 5. American Lung Association, New York, 1976.

Hinshaw, H. C., and Garland, L. H.: Diseases of the Chest, ed. 3. W. B. Saunders Company, Philadelphia, 1969.

Safar, P.: Respiratory Therapy. F. A. Davis Company, Philadelphia, 1965.

NOTES

NOTES

12

Metabolic and Respiratory Acidosis/Alkalosis: A Comparative Analysis

	METABOLIC ACIDOSIS	RESPIRATORY ACIDOSIS
DEFINITION:	Excess of acid (H^+) and deficit of base (HCO_3)	Excess of acid (H_2CO_3) and elevated pCO_2
PROBABLE CAUSE:	Ketoacidosis: incomplete metabolism of fats (diabetes); renal acidosis: retention of inorganic, phosphoric and sulfuric acids (renal failure); lactic acidosis: incomplete metabolism of CHO; HCO_3 deficit: diarrhea	Hypoventilation: retention of CO_2, i.e., COPD; muscular weakness
RECOGNITION:	Headache, nausea, vomiting, diarrhea, sensorium changes, tremoring, convulsions	Decreased ventilation, sensorium changes, somnolence, semicomatose-comatose, tachycardia, arrhythmia
LABORATORY TESTS:	pH<7.35 serum CO_2<22 mEq/L pCO_2<40 mmHg if compensating pO_2 usually normal serum K elevated	pH<7.35 serum CO_2>27 mEq/L if compensating pCO_2>40 mmHg pO_2 usually normal or low serum K elevated
SAMPLE LAB. TEST; UNCOMPENSATED:	pH 7.15 pCO_2 40 pO_2 88 HCO_3 8 (HCO_3/H_2CO_3 ratio is 8:1)	pH 7.15 pCO_2 60 pO_2 88 HCO_3 24 (HCO_3/H_2CO_3 ratio is 13:1)

SAMPLE LAB. TEST; COMPENSATED:	pH 7.35 pCO₂ 24 pO₂ 88 HCO₃ 8 (Lungs "blow off" pCO₂ by hyperventilation to decrease acids)	pH 7.35 pCO₂ 60 pO₂ 88 HCO₃ 39 (Kidneys hold HCO₃ to neutralize H₂CO₃)
TREATMENT:	Treat underlying cause; correct diabetic acidosis with glucose and insulin; rid body of excess protein and H⁺ ions with resins and/or dialysis; administer O₂, thereby encouraging CHO metabolism to CO₂ and H₂O; give NaHCO₃ intravenously.	Treat cause; improve ventilation by: IPPB, antibiotics, postural drainage, suction, endotracheal tube, tracheostomy, ventilator, NaHCO₃ (in emergency).
NURSE'S RESPONSIBILITIES:	Administer HCO₃; take seizure precautions; maintain intake-output record; fluid therapy, forced or restricted.	Improve ventilation by TCDB, semi-Fowler's position, low flow O₂; chest physiotherapy.
	METABOLIC ALKALOSIS	**RESPIRATORY ALKALOSIS**
DEFINITION:	Deficit of H⁺ and excess of Base (HCO₃)	Deficit of carbonic acid (H₂CO₃)
PROBABLE CAUSE:	Gastric losses via vomiting, stomach tube, lavage, potent diuretics.	Hyperventilation from neurogenic cause, brain trauma, ventilators.
RECOGNITION:	Nausea, vomiting, diarrhea, sensorium changes, tremoring, convulsions	Tachypnea, sensorium changes, numbness, tingling of hands and face
LABORATORY TESTS:	pH>7.45 serum CO₂>27 mEq/L pCO₂>40 if compensating pO₂ usually normal serum K decreased serum chloride decreased	pH>7.45 serum CO₂<22 mEq/L if compensating pCO₂<40 mmHg pO₂ usually normal serum K decreased urine alkaline
SAMPLE LAB. TEST; UNCOMPENSATED:	pH 7.52 pCO₂ 40 pO₂ 88 HCO₃ 36 (HCO₃/H₂CO₃ ratio is 30:1)	pH 7.52 pCO₂ 24 pO₂ 88 HCO₃ 24 (HCO₃/H₂CO₃ ratio is 40:1)

SAMPLE LAB. TEST; COMPENSATED:	pH 7.45 pCO_2 55 pO_2 88 HCO_3 36 (lungs retain CO_2 by hypoventilation to increase acids)	pH 7.45 pCO_2 24 pO_2 88 HCO_3 15 (kidneys excrete HCO_3 and retain H^+ ions)
TREATMENT:	Replace loss of fluids, especially K and Cl; administer acidifying IV fluid, e.g., ammonium Cl	Sedation, voluntary breath holding
NURSE'S RESPONSIBILITIES:	Maintain intake-output record; take seizure precautions; administer medications.	Give reassurance; encourage breathing into paper bag.

112

NOTES

SECTION V

CLINICAL SITUATIONS

13

Respiratory Diseases

This discussion of respiratory diseases is included because respiration is one of the primary regulators of fluid and electrolyte homeostasis. How changes in respiration affect the acid-base balance has already been discussed (see Chapter 11). This chapter will outline the respiratory problems which most frequently occur in the clinical situation.

Physiology

An understanding of the physiology of respiration and the anatomy of the respiratory system is necessary to enable the nurse to competently cope with respiratory problems that affect acid-base balance.

In normal respiration, air is inhaled through the external respiratory tract and drawn through the bronchial tree to the alveolar level where the exchange of gases occurs (Fig. 13-1). Respiration can be divided into three interdependent processes: alveolar ventilation, alveolar-capillary diffusion, and perfusion. Alveolar ventilation is the process by which atmospheric gases move in to the **alveoli.** Alveolar-capillary diffusion is the passage of alveolar gases into the arterial-capillary to be exchanged with venous gases across the thin alveolar-capillary membrane. Perfusion is the circulation of oxygenated blood through the alveolar-capillary membrane; then from the lungs to the tissues, and the subsequent inundation of the body cells with oxygenated blood.

The anatomy of the respiratory system influences the efficiency of respiration. The amount of air inhaled and exhaled in quiet breathing averages about 500 to 600 cc and is called the **tidal volume.** Any variation in the tidal volume will be reflected by a change in alveolar ventilation and a subsequent change in the entire respiratory process.

The alveoli are the functional units of the respiratory system. Most of the anatomy of the respiratory system is composed of passive airways which are referred to as anatomical dead space because the air does not participate in the exchange of gases in the passageways. Dead space includes the nasopharynx, the larynx, the trachea, and the main bronchi.

The numerous factors involved in the control of respiration include the carbon dioxide concentration, the hydrogen ion concentration (pH), the chemoreceptor system (oxygen deficiency), exercise, arterial pressure, sensory impulses, and speech. This concept of respiratory control is called the multiple factor theory.

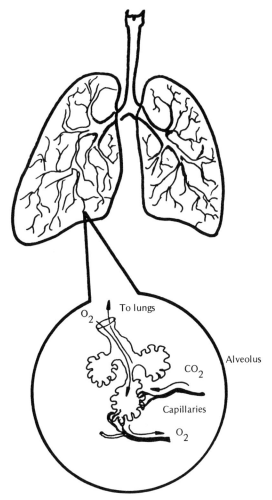

Figure 13-1.   Cross-section of lung with enlargement of alveolus.

Classification

Respiratory diseases, as well as various neuromuscular diseases, interrupt the normal respiratory cycle. Respiratory diseases may be classified as chronic or acute and as reversible or irreversible. Among the more common causes of chronic respiratory diseases are smoking, allergies, and chronic infections. Acute respiratory diseases may be caused by infection, tumors, atelectasis, obstruction, and chest trauma. Reversible respiratory diseases are those involving infections, edema, bronchial spasms, and obstruction. Irreversible respiratory diseases are those in which permanent destruction has occurred; these include emphysema, cancerous tumors, and infiltrative diseases.

Chronic Respiratory Diseases. Smoking is probably the greatest factor in chronic respiratory disease, since it is thought to be a major factor in cancer of the lung. Although smoking is not considered a direct cause of emphysema, there is a definite correlation between heavy smoking and emphysema. Air pollution has recently been recognized as another causative factor in res-

TABLE 13-1. CHRONIC RESPIRATORY DISEASE

Disease	Description	Recognition	Laboratory Tests	Treatment
Bronchitis ("blue bloater")	Inflammatory and/or infectious disease with airway obstruction; person has normal lung volume, is usually a smoker; closely related to emphysema	Productive cough; cyanosis; "puffiness"; cardiac involvement (cor pulmonale); CO_2 narcosis	Increased hemoglobin; increased hematocrit	Decrease smoking; antibiotics; **IPPB**; expectorants; humidification
Emphysema ("pink puffer")	Primarily exhalation problem; lung capacity increased; residual volume increased; elasticity decreased; alveolar damage; airway obstruction	Respiration labored; barrel-chested; weight loss; cor pulmonale	pCO_2 increased; globulin deficiency in blood	Bronchodilators; IPPB; tranquilizers; control infection; stop smoking; sodium restriction; diuretics
Pulmonary fibrosis	Ventilation and diffusion dysfunction; total lung capacity decreased	Dyspnea; cyanosis; clubbing of fingers; cor pulmonale; hyperventilation	pO_2 decreased; pCO_2 decreased (diagnosed by lung tissue biopsy)	Corticosteroids

TABLE 13-2. ACUTE RESPIRATORY DISEASES

Disease	Description	Recognition	Laboratory Tests	Treatment
Bronchial asthma	Acute airway obstruction due to allergic/nervous response; little or no hypoxemia	Respiratory distress; wheezing	CO_2 usually normal; O_2 decreased	Medication (adrenalin); IPPB; expectorants; bronchodilators
Bronchitis	Airway obstruction due to edema secondary to inflammation	Fever; chest pain; dyspnea; cough	White blood cell count (WBC) increased	Antibiotics; IPPB; expectorants; humidification
Pneumonia	Pneumococci; bacterial pathogens; gram negative bacilli; Staphylococcus aureus	Fever; productive cough; pulmonary infiltration	WBC increased; pO_2 decreased; pCO_2 may be increased	Antibiotics; IPPB; expectorants; humidification; hydration to thin secretions
Pulmonary edema	Acute heart failure; hypernatremia and fluid retention	Edema; weight gain; hypertension; dyspnea	Urine Cl decreased; serum sodium normal; hemoglobin normal or decreased	Diuretics; salt and fluid restriction
Pulmonary emboli	Capillaries plugged with clots	Chest pain; increased blood pressure	Lactic/dehydrogenase (LDH) increased	Anticoagulants
Respiratory depression	Insensitive respiratory center; sometimes accompanies obesity	CO_2 narcosis	pO_2 decreased; pCO_2 increased	Endotracheal tube; supportive breathing; respiratory stimulants
Spontaneous pneumothorax	Ruptured lung	Blood pressure and pulse decreased; movement of chest wall decreased; cyanosis	Xray	Release air by inserting catheter into intrapleural space through second intercostal space anteriorly; prophylactic antibiotics

piratory diseases. It is a source of aggravation to patients with chronic obstructive pulmonary disease **(COPD).**

Because emphysema is so common it is discussed here as well as in Table 13-1. Emphysema is a destructive, irreversible process. There is a ventilation defect in which the total lung capacity and the residual volume are increased. The primary difficulty in emphysema is in exhalation, as shown by the elevated pCO_2 reading. Diffusion is also a problem in that there is insufficient capillary surface through which blood gases may be exchanged. This may result from the presence of excessive fluids leading to an obstruction. The elasticity of the lung is decreased and the alveoli are gradually damaged. Emphysema is a chronic condition that can easily precipitate into an acute respiratory failure. In some cases, even the infectious process of a common cold can tip the scale toward acute respiratory failure.

Table 13-1 summarizes chronic respiratory diseases.

Acute Respiratory Diseases. Pneumonia, the most deadly of the acute infectious respiratory diseases, is the fifth most common cause of death in the United States today. Acute pneumonia is an infectious process caused by bacterial and viral pathogens. Pneumococcus appears to be the most frequent bacterial source, followed by the gram negative bacilli and Staphylococcus aureus. The tissues and the air spaces of the lungs become filled with fluid due to the inflammation usually caused by these bacteria.

Table 13-2 summarizes acute respiratory diseases.

The most common causes of death in acute respiratory failure are sedation (including aspirin), infection, inhalers (overuse causes arrhythmia), digitalis preparations, and electrolyte imbalance. Digitalis is often administered for **cor pulmonale;** however, the basic problem is the lung disease. Thus it would usually be preferable to treat the lung disease as well as the heart problem.

Nurse's Responsibilities

Evaluate ventilation.

Keep sedatives to a minimum.

Maintain low flow oxygen (1 to 2 L) in patients with chronic pulmonary diseases.

Be aware that chronic obstructive pulmonary disease can precipitate into acute respiratory failure from infection, congestive heart failure, drugs, atelectasis, or bronchitis.

Be alert to a decrease in aeration, an increase in pulse rate, restlessness, sweating, sensorium changes, and somnolence.

Keep airway free of secretions by encouraging coughing or by suctioning as necessary.

BIBLIOGRAPHY

Bates, D. V., Macklem, P. T., and Christie, R. V.: Respiratory Function in Disease, ed. 2. W. B. Saunders Company, Philadelphia, 1971.

Chronic Obstructive Pulmonary Disease, ed. 5. American Lung Association, New York, 1976.

Condon, R. E., and Nyhus, L. M.: Manual of Surgical Therapeutics, ed. 3. Little, Brown and Company, Boston, 1975.

Cotes, J. E.: Lung Function: Assessment and Application in Medicine, ed. 3. J. B. Lippincott Company, Philadelphia, 1975.

Gaensler, E. A.: Clinical pulmonary physiology. N. Engl. J. Med. 252:177, 221, 264, 1955.

Guyton, A. C.: Function of the Human Body, ed. 4. W. B. Saunders Company, Philadelphia, 1974.

Hinshaw, H. C., and Garland, L. H.: Diseases of the Chest, ed. 3. W. B. Saunders Company, Philadelphia, 1969.

Introduction to Lung Diseases, ed. 6. American Lung Association, New York, 1975.

MacKenzie, A. I., and Patterson, W. D.: Bilateral tension pneumothorax occurring during operation. Br. J. Anaesth. 43:987, 1971.

Price, J. D., and Lauerner, R. W.: Serum urine osmalities in the differential diagnosis of polyuric states. J. Clin. Endocrinol. Metab. 26:143, 1966.

Slonim, N. B., and Chapin, J. L.: Respiratory Physiology, ed. 2. The C. V. Mosby Company, St. Louis, 1971.

Spontaneous pneumothorax and apical lung disease. Br. Med. J. 4:573, 1971.

NOTES

NOTES

14

Acute Renal Failure

Acute renal failure is a condition in which renal function rapidly becomes impaired or ceases. Acute renal failure has been called the "$7,000 disease" because currently this is the average cost to the patient from onset to recovery.

An alert nurse can help prevent the development of acute renal failure. In most cases, the earliest sign of impending renal failure is a decrease in the urinary output. Nitrogenous waste products accumulate rapidly in the blood and the patient develops **azotemia.** This trend can be reversed in many instances by prompt and adequate treatment.

Physiology

The **nephron** is the functional unit of the kidney (Fig. 14-1). There are approximately three million of these microscopic units located in the curved outer part of the kidneys. The nephron contains the glomerulus (located inside the Bowman's capsule), the proximal convoluted tubules, the loop of Henle, and the distal convoluted tubules. About 25 per cent of the blood pumped by the heart passes through the kidneys. The kidneys filter approximately 160 to 170 liters of blood each 24 hours. One to one and one-half liters of fluid are extracted from the blood and concentrated into urine.

The normal kidneys regulate the volume and composition of the blood by filtration, selective reabsorption, and secretion. Filtration of the plasma takes place in the glomerulus where the fluid and dissolved substances are filtered through the capillary walls, the basement membrane, and the visceral layer of the Bowman's capsule. Glomerular filtrate, the product of this process, is a plasma-like substance minus protein and cells.

As the glomerular filtrate passes through the renal proximal tubules, selective reabsorption into the capillaries takes place. The proximal tubules reabsorb potassium, sodium, glucose, amino acids, and uric acid. Acid-base balance is partially regulated by the proximal tubules by the reabsorption or filtration of bicarbonate according to the body's needs.

Secretion takes place in the distal tubules. Hydrogen ions, potassium, and uric acid are secreted into the tubular fluid.

When kidney disease interrupts this regulation process, the filtrate is reabsorbed out of the tubules into the blood, taking water, electrolytes, and the nonvolatile products of metabolism with it. If this process is allowed to continue, death will result.

123

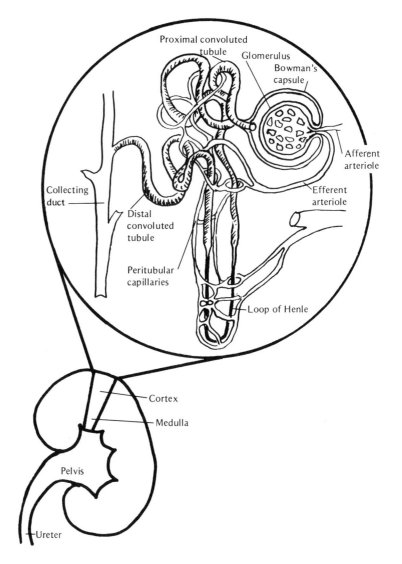

Figure 14-1.   Nephron.

Renal failure can be divided into three categories: prerenal, postrenal, and intrarenal (Fig. 14-2). Prerenal failure is caused by events that take place before the blood reaches the kidneys, and involves the subsequent reaction of normal kidneys to these stimuli. Postrenal failure may result from an obstruction in the system which leads away from the kidney. The third type, intrarenal failure, may be due to primary parenchymal damage, or it may be a sequela of pre- or postrenal failure.

Prerenal Failure

Table 14-1 lists the causes and altered functions of prerenal failure.

Recognition. The professional nurse should be alert to a decrease in urinary output. He should be aware of conditions that predispose the patient to oliguria; these conditions include intracellular and extracellular fluid deple-

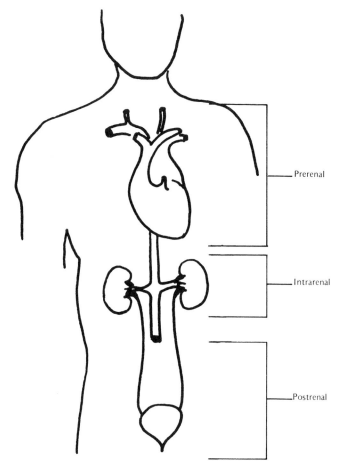

Figure 14-2.   Types of renal failure.

tion, diabetic acidosis, shock, and cardiac failure. Other visible signs or symptoms of prerenal failure are rare.

TABLE 14-1. CAUSES AND ALTERED FUNCTIONS OF PRERENAL FAILURE

Cause	*Altered Function*
Hypovolemia	Decreased fluid volume reduces renal blood flow and glomerular filtration rate
Decreased cardiac output	Kidneys not receiving the normal cardiac output (N25% of the body's blood)

Vascular failure
   vasogenic shock
   neurogenic shock
	Interference with vascular elasticity by vascular collapse or pooling of the blood (vascular dilation)

Hepatorenal syndrome	Diseased liver causes body to falsely sense a volume deficit, thus retaining fluids; liver becomes grossly edematous

Laboratory Tests. BUN and creatinine levels are elevated with a 20:1 or greater ratio, respectively. Specific gravity is usually greater than 1.020 because the kidneys are trying to concentrate the urine. The urine sodium level will be less than 20 mEq/L. It may drop much lower than 20 mEq/L if the patient has a saline deficit, because the kidneys will retain sodium in the serum. Urine osmolality will be above 450 **mOsm**/kg and is usually greater than plasma osmolality.

Treatment. The treatment of prerenal failure is aimed at restoring adequate circulation to the kidneys and correcting the underlying cause.

Mannitol, an osmotic diuretic, may be administered intravenously to determine whether the condition is prerenal or intrarenal failure. Mannitol is both a diagnostic aid and a temporary treatment. If the condition is prerenal, there should be an adequate increase in urine output within three hours. If a fluid deficit is thought to be the cause of the prerenal failure, 1500 cc of 5 per cent dextrose in half-strength normal saline solution, lactated Ringer's solution, or normal saline solution may be given intravenously. If fluid deficit is the cause, the urine flow will increase.

Nurse's Responsibilities. The nurse will probably be the first member of the health team to become aware of a decrease in the urinary output. At the first suspicion of urinary decrease, the nurse should measure urinary output hourly with a urometer. The physician should be notified immediately if oliguria exists or is developing. The nurse's prompt report to the physician and immediate execution of his orders may prevent the development of acute renal failure.

When an oliguric condition exists, the nurse should assume the following responsibilities:

Observe for changes in vital signs.
Observe for fluid overload.
Observe for extracellular fluid excess.
Decrease the patient's potassium intake.
Maintain accurate intake-output records.

Postrenal Failure

Table 14-2 identifies the causes and altered functions of postrenal failure.

TABLE 14-2. CAUSES AND ALTERED FUNCTIONS OF POSTRENAL FAILURE

Cause	Altered Function
Urethral obstruction (prostatism, tumors)	Complete obstruction causes anuria; partial obstruction usually causes anuria alternating with polyuria
Ureteral obstruction (calculi, tumors, trauma)	Complete obstruction causes anuria; partial obstruction usually causes anuria alternating with polyuria; edema following instrumentation
Sulfa or urate precipitation	Blockage due to precipitation or crystal formation
Anticholinergic drugs and ganglionic blocking agents	Acute urinary retention possible because nerves not adequately stimulated; however, this is unusual.

Recognition. With postrenal failure, the patient becomes **anuric** (less than 10 cc urine output in 24 hours). When only a partial obstruction exists, anuria will alternate with polyuria. Diuresis will follow the release of the obstruction.

Laboratory Tests. Urinalysis may reveal scanty sediment, occasional white and red blood cells, and hyaline or finely granular casts.

X rays may be taken to assess kidney size and to determine if renal stones or obstructions are present.

Treatment. The treatment is to relieve the obstruction.

Nurses' Responsibilities. Nursing care is similar to that practiced for other types of renal failure.

Report anuria to physician immediately.

Report pain to physician, as this can aid in diagnosis.

Check for fluid and electrolyte depletion during diuresis.

Maintain accurate intake-output records.

Intrarenal Failure

Table 14-3 identifies the causes and altered functions of intrarenal failure.

Recognition. Decreased urinary output or oliguria exists. As an azotemic condition develops, so do central nervous system symptoms.

Intracellular and extracellular fluid depletion, diabetic acidosis, shock, and cardiac failure are predisposing conditions to acute renal failure.

There are few visible signs. The most significant indicators are changes in urinary output and laboratory tests.

Laboratory Tests. Laboratory tests can be very significant in diagnosing acute renal failure. The BUN and creatinine levels are elevated. When oliguria is present, the BUN reading will rise approximately 20 points or more per day (as in sepsis). A creatinine clearance test will often show a marked decrease before BUN and creatinine levels show significant elevation.

The specific gravity of the urine is less than 1.015. Urine osmolality is below 450 mOsm/kg and is less than or near plasma osmolality. The urine sodium is above 40 mEq/L because the kidney is not able to reabsorb sodium.

The ratio of urine urea nitrogen to BUN and of urine creatinine concentration to plasma creatinine concentration is less than 10 to 1.

In acute tubular necrosis, the urinalysis shows the presence of renal tubular cells, tubular cell casts, coarsely granular casts, red blood cells, and hemoglobin, and red blood cell casts. In acute glomerulonephritis, urinalysis shows hematuria, proteinuria, and the presence of red blood cell and hemoglobin casts.

Treatment. Acute renal failure is a condition of parenchymal damage that is temporarily irreversible. Treatment is designed to maintain the patient until the acute lesion is healed and normal renal function resumes.

In acute renal failure, the oliguric phase usually lasts ten days to three weeks. Fluid intake should be carefully regulated during this period. Fluid allowance is calculated on the basis of 800 cc for insensible loss (800 cc/day), minus the amount acquired from **catabolism** (approximately 400 cc). Thus the fluid allowance is about 400 cc per 24 hours. The amount of fluid allowed for insensible loss may vary according to the amount lost through diaphoresis and the gastrointestinal tract. The restriction of fluid is essential to prevent a fluid excess and the consequent possibility of congestive heart failure and pulmonary edema.

Because it is difficult to provide sufficient calories, a 20 to 50 per cent glucose solution is often administered to supply 100 to 200 grams of sugar

TABLE 14-3. CAUSES AND ALTERED FUNCTIONS OF INTRARENAL FAILURE

Cause	*Altered Function*
Acute tubular necrosis	
Ischemia	Shock decreases renal perfusion causing circulatory insufficiency; resultant hypoxia causes tissue death
Drugs, poisons, metals	Nephrotoxic substances cause tissue injury and scarring
Hemolysis	Mismatched blood transfusion causes agglutination of red blood cells which obstruct tubules
Hypercalcemic crisis	Excess calcium crystallizes in tubules causing obstruction; condition varies according to pH of urine
Trauma	Burns and crushing injuries result in ECF deficit causing insufficient tissue perfusion; myoglobin causes sludging in tubules
Acute glomerulonephritis	
Post-streptococcal infection	Antigen-antibody reaction in glomerulus causes inflammation and decreased glomerular blood flow
Vascular	
Renal arterial thrombosis	Thrombi in renal vessels cause occlusion
Acute cortical necrosis	
Pregnancy (abruptio placenta)	Intravascular coagulation possibly due to amniotic fluid in the plasma; anuria without obstruction
Sepsis (especially in pregnant women and patients on steroid therapy)	White blood cells fail to handle toxins as they would under normal conditions
Papillary necrosis	
Urinary tract infection	Papillae sluff off; particles obstruct the tubules
Intrarenal precipitation	
Urates and sulfonamides	Precipitation and crystal formation cause obstruction
Multiple myeloma	Precipitation of myeloma protein into kidney
Pyelonephritis	Infection of kidney causes scarring of tubular system

daily. Sodium is usually not administered unless a deficit exists or excessive losses occur through diaphoresis or the gastrointestinal tract.

Potassium is not administered because acute renal failure increases the likelihood of hyperkalemia, which may result in cardiac arrest. Although there is no potassium intake, tissue catabolism increases the serum potassium level. Acute and severe hyperkalemia can be effectively treated by intravenous infusion of sodium bicarbonate, calcium gluconate, or glucose and insulin. Kayexalate, a cation-exchange ion, given orally or rectally, is also effective but acts more slowly. In order to limit urea in the serum, protein is severely limited or omitted from the diet.

Renal acidosis will develop because the kidneys are unable to excrete the 50 to 70 mEq of nonvolatile acids produced daily. Peritoneal dialysis or hemodialysis may be used to alleviate the uremia if other methods are inadequate.

Blood transfusions are often necessary in acute renal failure. Whole fresh blood should be used because cell breakdown causes a higher potassium content in stored blood. Anemia develops in 10 to 14 days following the onset of acute renal failure.

Anabolic steroids, such as testosterone propionate in oil, may be administered to decrease protein catabolism.

One of the primary causes of death in acute renal failure is the patient's susceptibility to infection; for this reason, indwelling catheters are seldom inserted. Because many antibiotics are excreted through the kidneys, the amount administered should be reduced during acute renal failure. Some antibiotics, though not all, can cause nephrotoxicity in acute renal failure. Penicillin is nontoxic and can be administered in normal dosages. Tetracycline should be avoided because its action enhances catabolism and causes the BUN level to rise. Mandelamine and NegGram should not be used. Kanamycin Sulfate, Polymyxin, and Garamycin are usually given only every two or three days. Keflin and Cephaloridine should also be reduced. Antibiotic levels in the blood must be determined; antibiotics may have to be reduced or discontinued due to nephrotoxicity. The length of time that the antibiotic is retained in the blood can be determined by using the following formula:

serum creatinine level X 4 = number of hours antibiotic retained

Thus, if the serum creatinine level is six (6 x 4 = 24 hours), the antibiotic will be retained in the blood for 24 hours. All patients who receive nephrotoxic antibiotics for over one week should be monitored with a 24-hour creatinine clearance test.

Nurse's Responsibilities. Maintain accurate intake-output records.

Accurately measure body weight.

Practice medical asepsis.

Encourage coughing and deep breathing.

Assist with mouth care: teeth should be brushed and an antiseptic mouth wash used at least every two hours.

Assist with emotional/mental needs.

The prolonged stress of acute renal failure may lead to psychotic behavior; this possibility usually increases when the patient is in reverse isolation. Helping the patient to cope with confusion and restlessness presents an additional nursing care challenge. Avoid oversedation because many sedatives and tranquilizers are excreted through the kidneys. A pleasant atmosphere, radio and television, and current news may help the patient remain oriented to reality during this stress situation.

Conclusion

If renal failure is successfully reversed, recovery of renal function usually begins within 10 to 14 days. Urine volume increases progressively to normal or polyuria within a few days, but complete recovery of function may take several weeks. (Some patients do not attain complete recovery, because their creatinine levels remain increased.) During the diuretic phase, polyuria may develop because the convalescing kidneys cannot yet conserve sodium and water, and urea is not excreted efficiently. As a result, the BUN level may remain elevated, and the excess urea will act as a diuretic. The excessive fluid loss may deplete the extracellular volume to such an extent that shock develops. During the diuretic phase, when there is danger of severe electrolyte depletion, the patient should be monitored. All fluid loss should *not* be replaced, because excessive administration of fluids prolongs polyuria.

The cause of death in acute renal failure is usually the primary trauma or disease, fluid excess, infection, or hyperkalemia. The mortality rate is approximately 40 per cent. Incomplete recovery from acute renal failure can lead to chronic renal disease.

CASE STUDY
14*

A 50-year-old woman was transferred to an intensive care unit four days after receiving a mismatched blood transfusion. Upon admission, she was oliguric with a urinary output of 200 cc/24 hours, her BUN reading was 96 mg %, and serum creatinine was 8 mg %. Admission urinalysis showed a sp gr of 1.012 and a urinary sodium level of 50 mEq/L.

Her BUN/creatinine levels continued to rise daily. With the azotemia, she developed central nervous system symptoms. Following the diagnosis of acute renal failure, she was taken to surgery for the insertion of a shunt, preparatory to hemodialysis therapy.

At the time of the first hemodialysis treatment, the BUN was 148 mg %, serum creatinine 15 mg %, and potassium 6.8 mEq/L. She was placed on a cardiac monitor, and her fluids and diet were carefully regulated.

Within the next two weeks anemia developed (Hgb 9 gms), and she was treated with fresh packed cells. The hemodialysis treatments continued as indicated for the next three weeks, at which time normal kidney function began to return.

Questions

1. How does a mismatched blood transfusion cause acute renal failure?

2. Why is the urinary sodium level elevated?

3. Why was the patient placed on a cardiac monitor?

---

*For answers to Case Study Questions, see Appendix 4.

4. Discuss the probable fluid and diet regime for this patient.

5. Why was the patient given *fresh* packed cells to treat the anemia?

Case Summary: This patient developed severe psychotic problems which took many months to resolve. Her recovery from the renal failure was slow; it was about one and one-half years before the BUN level returned to normal.

Quiz 14*

A 50-year-old woman was transferred to an intensive care unit following a mismatched blood transfusion and subsequent development of acute renal failure.

Check the following as true or false:

True	False		
_____	_____	1.	Accurate body weight measurements are extremely important when a patient is on hemodialysis.
_____	_____	2.	H₂O is given more freely when a patient is on hemodialysis.
_____	_____	3.	During the diuretic phase, all fluids lost should be replaced.
_____	_____	4.	Hyperkalemia causes tachycardia.
_____	_____	5.	Catabolism is the same as oxidation.
_____	_____	6.	BUN rises 20 points or more daily in acute renal failure.
_____	_____	7.	Acidosis is never a problem in acute renal failure.
_____	_____	8.	A catheter is always left in place during acute renal failure.
_____	_____	9.	Patients with acute renal failure are susceptible to infection.
_____	_____	10.	The immediate administration of Mannitol might have prevented the development of acute renal failure.

BIBLIOGRAPHY

Davidson, R.C., and Scribner, B. H.: A Physician's Syllabus for the Treatment of Chronic Uremia. University of Washington, Seattle, 1967.

Flinn, R. B., Merrill, J. P., and Welzant, W. R.: Treatment of the oliguric patient with a new sodium-exchange resin and sorbitol: A preliminary report. New Eng. J. Med. 264:111, 1960.

---

*For answers to Quizzes, see Appendix 5.

Franklin, S. S., and Merrill, J. P.: Acute renal failure. N. Engl. J. Med. 292:711, 1960.

Holland, P. V., and Wallerstein, R. O.: Delayed hemolytic transfusion reaction with acute renal failure. J.A.M.A. 204:1007, 1968.

Levinsky, N. G.: Acute renal failure. N. Engl. J. Med. 274: 1016, 1966.

Maher, J. F., and Schreiner, G. E.: Hazards and complications of dialysis. N. Engl. J. Med. 273:370, 1965.

Merrill, J. P.: Kidney disease: Acute renal failure. Annu. Rev. Med. 11:127, 1960.

Merrill, J. P.: The Treatment of Renal Failure, ed. 2. Grune & Stratton, Inc., New York, 1965.

Oken, D. E.: Diagnosis and treatment of acute renal failure. Mod. Treat. 6:927, 1969.

Papper, Solomon: Clinical Nephrology. Little, Brown and Company, Boston, 1971.

Perillie, P. B., and Conn, H. O.: Acute renal failure after intravenous pyelography in plasma cell myeloma. J.A.M.A. 167:2186, 1958.

Porter, R., and Knight, J.: Energy Metabolism in Trauma. CIBA Foundation, Churchhill, London, 1970.

Ravel, R.: Clinical Laboratory Medicine. Year Book Medical Publishers, Inc., Chicago, 1970.

NOTES

NOTES

15

Chronic Renal Failure

Chronic renal insufficiency is often asymptomatic until it is manifested by its complications. A 75 per cent deterioration in the reserve function of the kidneys can occur before identifiable symptoms appear. The condition progresses gradually and causes varying degrees of irreversible damage to the kidneys, making them unable to filter all the waste products from the blood, especially protein by-products. The disease usually damages the nephrons, decreasing or destroying the glomerular or tubular function. Most commonly the damage is caused by four factors: antigen-antibody deposits in the glomerular basement membrane (lupus erythematosus, post-streptococcal glomerulonephritis); thickening or occlusion of arterioles (nephrosclerosis); obstructive substances (calcium deposits or uric acid); and scarring due to necrosis and infection (pyelonephritis).

Causes

Table 15-1 lists the causes and altered functions of chronic renal insufficiency.

Complications

Although chronic renal failure is a disease of the kidneys, almost every other area of the body becomes affected. These complications must be treated as they appear. Table 15-2 lists the more common complications.

Recognition

Chronic renal disease is usually well advanced before it is recognized. Its signs and symptoms are also indicative of other disease processes.

Symptoms include loss of appetite, headache, nausea, vomiting, and itching. Polyuria accompanied by **isosthenuria,** nocturia, oliguria, and **polydipsia** may appear. Recognizable signs include a sallow complexion, listlessness, edema, peripheral neuropathy (foot drop, loss of ankle jerk), elevated blood pressure, and uremic frost caused by perspiration and uric acid.

The patient may develop renal metabolic acidosis, and hyperventilation may be present.

Laboratory Tests

Laboratory tests will indicate elevated BUN and creatinine levels. The

TABLE 15-1. CAUSES AND ALTERED FUNCTIONS OF
CHRONIC RENAL INSUFFICIENCY

Cause	Altered Function
Glomerulonephritis	
Proliferative	Diffuse increased cellularity of glomeruli; lesions due to antigen-antibody reaction; inflamation and dysfunction of glomerulus; most commonly seen in post-streptococcal glomerulonephritis; frequently a recoverable lesion
Membranous	Thickening of the basement membrane; usually idiopathic (also seen in diabetic renal disease); leads to heavy loss of protein; nephrotic state
Focal	Non-diffuse scattered lesions of proliferative, membranous, or membranous-proliferative type; frequently benign; most common symptom is hematuria
Nephrosclerosis	Hardening of renal tissues resulting in narrowing or occlusion of vessels; arteriosclerosis related to aging process which is accelerated in uncontrolled hypertension
Pyelonephritis	Kidney damage attributed to chronic infection with micro-organisms beginning in the renal pelvis and proceeding to renal parenchyma
Papillary necrosis	Obstruction and sloughing of the papillae may be related to diabetes, infection, analgesic drug abuse, urinary obstruction
Uric acid nephropathy	Uric acid causes blockage of tubules
Nephrocalcinosis	High concentration of calcium in the blood causes calcium deposits with subsequent renal damage; seen in many diseases, such as hyperparathyroidism and sarcoidosis
Lupus erythematosus	A collagen-vascular disease; no set pattern of events; renal involvement most often focal but can cause proliferative or membranous glomerulonephritis
Acute renal failure	Incomplete recovery can lead to chronic renal failure
Sickle cell anemia	Hereditary "S" shaped hemoglobin cells cause sloughing into and plugging of the glomeruli; significant to the Negroid race
Polycystic kidney disease	Congenital hereditary disease causes formation of cysts whose enlargement causes pressure and atrophy of functioning glomeruli

TABLE 15-2. COMPLICATIONS OF CHRONIC RENAL FAILURE
AND THEIR LOCATION

Location	Complication
Cranial	Decreased mental alertness; impaired vision and hearing; glossitis; parotitis
Thoracic	Infection (pneumonia, pleurisy); fluid retention (pulmonary edema)
Cardiovascular	Congestive heart failure; uremic pericarditis; hypertension (ECF increased); arrhythmias (elevated potassium in terminal stages)
Gastrointestinal	Nausea, vomiting; hematemesis, paralytic ileus, melena
Reproductive	Decreased ovulation or spermatogenesis; vaginal hemorrhage; impotence
Skeletal	Osteodystrophy due to secondary hypertrophy of parathyroid glands; this causes increased vascular and extraskeletal calcifications; hypertrophy of parathyroid glands occurs because the body is attempting, without success, to keep the serum Ca and PO_4 normal
Integumentary	Itching due to microscopic Ca and PO_4 deposits in the skin caused by overactive parathyroid glands
Hemal	Anemia due to three factors: decreased erythropoietin (a hormone produced by the kidneys that stimulates the bone marrow); shorter life span of red cells due to uremic factors of hemolysis in the blood; oozing blood through the bowels
Neural	Tingling; numbness (blood supply to nerves decreased); seizures (high BUN toxic to central nervous system); sensorium changes (ICF excess); hyperreflexia; asterixis

serum creatinine-creatinine clearance test is the best single measurement of renal function. The 24-hour test is essential. For an accurate test, the nurse must report, to the minute, the exact time the test begins and ends. The following formula indicates why this accuracy is so important:

$$\frac{\text{urine creatinine}}{\text{serum creatinine}} \times \frac{\text{urine volume}}{\text{minutes}} \times \frac{1.73}{\text{area}} = \begin{array}{l}\text{blood (cc) cleared of} \\ \text{creatinine per minute} \\ \text{(glomerular filtration} \\ \text{rate)}\end{array}$$

Normal creatinine clearance is 100 to 130 cc per minute.

Other tests may indicate normochromic anemia, renal acidosis, calcium decreased, phosphorous increased, and serum sodium decreased. Fasting blood sugar is often elevated and the glucose tolerance test may be abnormal. If so, the patient is not necessarily diabetic. A urinalysis will show a fixed specific gravity of 1.010 to 1.015, indicating an inability to concentrate and dilute urine. An albumin level elevation of 1 to 4+ in the urine suggests damage to the filtering system of the glomerulus. The urine may also contain red blood cells, bacteria, and casts.

In the terminal stages the potassium level may increase and result in EKG changes showing elevated T waves.

Treatment

The goal in the treatment of chronic renal failure is to assist the patient to maintain optimal renal function. The patient will generally respond well if he adheres to the treatment plan.

Chronic renal failure is usually controlled conservatively with proper diet and fluid restriction. A low protein and high caloric diet is used most frequently. Sodium is usually restricted since about 80 per cent of these patients retain salt. The remaining 20 per cent lose salt. If the urine sodium level is *below* 20 mEq/L, the patient will usually be considered a salt-retainer. If the urine sodium level is *over* 20 mEq/L, and if extracellular fluid depletion results in a postural blood pressure decrease while on a salt-restricted diet, the patient is a salt-loser. In her book, *Nutrition and Diet Therapy,* Sue Rodwell Williams states:

> The variables of treatment center primarily upon protein, sodium, potassium, and water. Levels of each nutrient will need to be individually adjusted according to progression of the illness, type of treatment being used, and the patient's response to treatment. In general, however, overall treatment has several basic objectives:
> 1) To reduce and minimize protein catabolism
> 2) To avoid . . . [ECF-ICF deficit or ECF-ICF excess]
> 3) To carefully correct acidosis
> 4) To correct electrolyte depletions and avoid excesses
> 5) To control fluid and electrolyte losses from vomiting and diarrhea
> 6) To maintain nutrition and weight
> 7) To maintain appetite and morale
> 8) To control complications such as hypertension, bone pain, and central nervous system abnormalities.*

Infections are treated with antibiotics. However, antibiotics should be used cautiously and only in appropriate dosages.

Increased phosphorous is treated with an antacid that does not contain magnesium.

In cases that do not respond to these conservative treatments, the more complex procedures of peritoneal dialysis (Chapter 20), hemodialysis (Chapter 21), and/or kidney transplants must be used.

Nurse's Responsibilities

When a patient with chronic renal disease is hospitalized, it is usually for diagnostic purposes, evaluation, complications, or treatment of unrelated diseases. Regardless of the reason, the nurse plays an important part in helping to maintain and manage the patient.

The responsibilities of the nurse include the following:
Maintain accurate intake-output records.
Take accurate daily weight measurements.
Implement diet restrictions.

---

*Sue Rodwell Williams: Nutrition and Diet Therapy, ed. 2. C. V. Mosby, St. Louis, 1973, pp. 556–557.

Calculate fluids as ordered.

Be alert to vital sign changes (elevated blood pressure, extracellular fluid excess, postural blood pressure changes).

Report abnormal electrolyte readings immediately.

Take seizure precautions.

Provide emotional support.

Be aware that a crisis situation could occur if any of the following problems develop: renal metabolic acidosis, hyperventilation, elevated potassium level resulting in EKG changes, oliguria, decreased calcium, elevated BUN and creatinine levels, and/or extracellular fluid excess.

CASE STUDY 15 *

A 46-year-old woman was admitted to the hospital for treatment of hypertension. She complained of not feeling well for the past year, and that she had grown progressively worse. In the past three months she had developed nausea, intermittent hematemesis, headache, weakness, poor appetite with a subsequent loss of 50 pounds. She further complained of itching, severe upper right quadrant pain, and cessation of menses. She appeared listless. Her blood pressure on admission was 182/104. She had no specific urinary symptoms other than occasional chills and fever.

Laboratory report: Hgb 7.3 gm %, HCT 22; BUN 165 Mg %; creatinine 16 mg %; Na 148 mEq/L; K 4.3 mEq/L; Cl 111 mEq/L; CO_2 12 mEq/L.

Urinalysis: 1-10 RBC; 1-8 WBC; 1-6 casts; 3+ albumin; bacteria.

Questions

1. This patient's signs and symptoms plus the laboratory reports are significant of what disease?

2. Evaluate the abnormal laboratory values.

3. What procedures can the nurse begin on her own initiative?

4. Explain the normal potassium reading in a patient with renal disease.

5. How will this patient's fluid intake be calculated?

6. Discuss diet requirements for patients with chronic renal disease.

Case Summary: A kidney biopsy revealed an idiopathic membranous glomerulonephritis. Because the disease was too advanced for conservative therapy, the patient was placed on hemodialysis therapy until a suitable donor could be found for a kidney transplant.

Quiz 15*

A 46-year-old woman was admitted to the hospital for treatment of hypertension. She complained of nausea, intermittent hematemesis, headache, general malaise, and poor appetite with weight loss. Among her laboratory reports were: Hgb 7.3 gm; BUN 165 mg %; creatinine 16 mg %; CO_2 12 mEq/L. Urinalysis: 1–6 casts, 3+ albumin.

1. What is hematemesis?

2. Serum CO_2 12, BUN 165 and creatinine 16 indicate a
   _____ acidosis.

3. Check the following true or false:

True	False	Patients with chronic renal disease:
_____	_____	a. are less alert as their condition deteriorates.
_____	_____	b. are prone to infection.
_____	_____	c. are in danger of developing uremic pericarditis.
_____	_____	d. often develop itching due to overactive parathyroid glands.
_____	_____	e. develop anemia due to decreased erythropoietin.
_____	_____	f. have a decreased blood supply to the nerves.

4. What is the best single test to measure renal function?

5. A patient with renal disease never has a normal potassium level.
   _____ True _____ False

6. A patient with chronic renal failure should be on a:
   _____ a. high protein, high caloric diet.
   _____ b. low protein, high caloric diet.
   _____ c. low protein, low caloric diet.
   _____ d. none of the above.

BIBLIOGRAPHY

Berman, L. B., and Schreiner, G. E.: Clinical and histologic spectrum of the nephrotic syndrome. Am. J. Med. 24:249, 1958.

*For answers to Quizzes, see Appendix 5.

Bland, J. H.: Clinical Metabolism of Body Water and Electrolytes. W. B. Saunders Company, Philadelphia, 1963, Chapter 2.

Brown, R.: Plasma erythropoietin in chronic uremia. Br. Med. J. 2:1036, 1965.

Churg, J., and Dolger, H.: Diabetic Renal Disease. In Strauss, M. B., and Welt, L. G. (eds.), Diseases of the Kidney, Vol. II, ed. 2. Little, Brown and Company, Boston, 1971.

CIBA: Chronic Renal Failure. Clin. Symp. Vol. 25, No. 1, 1973.

Dixon, F. J.: The pathogenesis of glomerulonephritis. Am. J. Med. 44:493, 1968.

Donodio, J. V.: Conservative management of chronic renal failure. Med. Clin. North Am. 50:1115, 1966.

Lee, L.: Antigen-antibody reaction in pathogenesis of bilateral renal cortical necrosis. J. Exp. Med. 117:365, 1963.

Levitsky, N. G.: Current concepts: Management of chronic renal failure. N. Eng. J. Med. 271:358, 1964.

Loge, J. P., Lange, R. D., and Moore, C. V.: Characterization of the anemia associated with chronic renal insufficiency. Am. J. Med. 24:4, 1958.

Maddick, R. K., Stevens, L. E., Reemstma, K., and Bloomer, H. A.: Goodpastures syndrome: Cessation of pulmonary hemorrhage after bilateral nephrectomy. Ann. Intern. Med. 67:1258, 1967

Merrill, J. P.: Management of chronic renal failure. Am. J. Med. 36:763, 1964.

Papper, S.: Clinical Nephrology. Little, Brown and Company, Boston, 1971.

Paton, R. R., Hegstrom, R. M., and Orme, B. M.: Fluid-Electrolyte Disorders. Mason Clinic, Seattle, 1969.

Schreiner, G. E.: The Nephrotic Syndrome. In Strauss, M. B., and Welt, L. G. (eds.), Diseases of the Kidney, Vol. II, ed. 2. Little, Brown and Company, Boston, 1971.

Williams, S. R.: Nutrition and Diet Therapy. The C. V. Mosby Company, St. Louis, 1973.

142

NOTES

16

Adrenal Disorders

The adrenal glands are involved in the regulation of selected electrolytes. Any change in the function of the adrenals will result in a change in the electrolyte balance. Of the two parts of the adrenals, the cortex is most important in the regulation of electrolytes. The anterior pituitary secretes a hormone called the adrenocorticotrophic hormone (ACTH) that stimulates the adrenal cortex to produce three groups of hormones: **glucocorticoids,** mineralcorticoids, and androgens, which are sex hormones. All of these hormones are steroids. The glucocorticoids are responsible primarily for converting starches, fats, and proteins into glucose, in that order. The mineralcorticoids, called the salt hormones, are responsible for helping to maintain blood pressure by retaining salt, and thus sodium, chloride, and water. They also cause a loss of potassium. The mineralcorticoids act upon the distal tubules of the kidneys. The sex hormones are not significant unless an abnormality exists. Normally, all three groups of adrenal hormones are secreted in stress response or in reaction to an altered function.

All of the above-mentioned hormones are related to the anterior pituitary. The posterior pituitary secretes an additional hormone, the antidiuretic hormone (ADH), that also acts upon the distal tubules of the kidney. ADH causes only the retention of water.

Pathology

An overproduction or underproduction of hormones by the adrenal glands will result in electrolyte and pH imbalances. The following overview classifies adrenal problems as related either to underproduction (hypoadrenalism) or to overproduction (hyperadrenalism):

Underproduction of hormones:
    acute failure with adrenal crisis, as in the Waterhouse-Friderichsen
        syndrome (meningococcal infection)
    chronic primary deficiency (Addison's disease)
    chronic secondary deficiency (pituitary hypofunction)
    hypoaldosteronism (lack of aldosterone)
Overproduction of hormones or their metabolites:
    Cushing's syndrome
    hyperaldosteronism

Adrenal Crisis

Adrenal crisis is usually a complication of a chronic deficiency and results when the adrenal glands are unable to cope with an increased stress situation superimposed on the chronic deficiency. Increased stress could be infection, colds, drugs, trauma, hemorrhage, or surgery. Any kind of stress requires increased secretion of hormones. In hypofunction, sufficient mineralcorticoids and glucocorticoids are not available to be secreted, even with increased stimulation. Crisis may also be induced by adrenalectomy, or by a too rapid withdrawal from prolonged treatment with steroids.

Recognition. The more common signs and symptoms include a slow development of weakness progressing to vascular insufficiency. Increased stress from a meningococcal infection may cause a severe hyperthermia to progress to hypothermia, coma, and shock. This type of crisis develops from the decreasing blood volume that results from the failure to retain sodium, chloride, and water. Thus, it actually leads to an extracellular volume deficit.

Laboratory Tests. The laboratory tests will show a reduced plasma cortisol level (cortisone) and a reduced aldosterone level because less hormones are produced. The urine should also be checked for the presence of electrolytes. The serum ratio of sodium to potassium in the urine is reduced.

Treatment. Treatment includes 100 mg intravenous administration of the hormones cortisol phosphate or succinate, repeated in doses of 50 mg every six hours. Treatment of shock, electrolyte deficits, and hypoglycemia may also be necessary. These problems may be counteracted by glucose, saline, and vasopressors, respectively. Infection may be the cause of the adrenal crisis and must be treated.

Chronic Deficiency (Addison's Disease)

Chronic deficiency, or Addison's disease, is a disease of the adrenal cortex resulting from a deficiency in the amount of corticosteroids produced over an extended period. Chronic deficiency, by strict definition, includes diseases of hypofunction restricted to the spontaneous and slower secretion of adrenal hormones. Hypofunction may be the result of destruction of the cortex by cancer metastasis, tuberculosis, fungus, infection, or atrophy of unknown origin. Chronic deficiency does not usually manifest itself until nine-tenths of the cortex is gone. A superimposed stress will produce temporary symptoms because of the increased need for the scantily available hormones. The disease is more common in adults, predominately occurring in the female. A possible hereditary tendency has been suggested.

Recognition. The cardinal symptoms of Addison's disease are increased pigmentation of the skin, physical and mental **asthenia** (easy fatigability), hypotension, and gastrointestinal disorders.

Increased pigmentation of the skin is due to excess ACTH and melanin stimulating hormone (MSH). Darkening of freckles and milk-white patches of skin surrounded by normal pigmentation are apparent. The skin may first have a dingy, smoky appearance that eventually progresses to a dark amber or bronze. Pigmentation changes are most marked in regions exposed to light and friction. The skin acquires the consistency of leather, and body hair usually decreases. These skin changes are seen only in chronic, not in acute deficiency. Table 16-1 categorizes by body system the basic signs and symptoms of hypoadrenalism.

Carbohydrate metabolism is affected and results in a decreased amount of glycogen stored in the liver. The patient will have fasting hypoglycemia; occasionally this is associated with diabetes mellitus.

TABLE 16-1. SIGNS AND SYMPTOMS OF CHRONIC PRIMARY
INSUFFICIENCY (HYPOADRENALISM)

System	Signs and Symptoms
Integumentary	Increased pigmentation due to excess ACTH and melanin stimulating hormone (MSH)
Central nervous	Personality disturbances such as listlessness, apathy, depression, irritability, and negativism, possibly progressing to psychosis; other possible symptoms include neuralgia, headache, vertigo, tinnitus, insomnia
Cardiovascular	Systolic/diastolic hypotension due to decrease in blood volume; small heart; orthostatic hypotension; circulatory collapse in crisis
Gastrointestinal	Anorexia; nausea, vomiting, diarrhea, occasional steatorrhea; weight loss; sensitivity to salt, sweet, bitter, and sour tastes
Reproductive	Decreased libido; menses usually normal

Laboratory Tests. The laboratory tests will show decreased sodium and chloride levels in the blood, with an increased potassium level. When deprived of salt in the diet, patients with Addison's disease lose sodium and chloride in the urine because the steroids needed for retention are not being adequately produced. Thus, the amount of sodium and chloride in the urine is increased, and the potassium is decreased. Metabolic acidosis is the pH imbalance associated with an increased potassium level. There is a correlation between increased BUN and a decreased extracellular fluid volume. Fasting hypoglycemia may be present because of the decreased glucocorticoids. Urinary studies may show decreased amounts of 17-ketosteroids, corticosteroids, and aldosterone.

When the production of steroids is decreased, the number of eosinophils, a type of white blood cell, will increase. When ACTH is given to a person with Addison's disease, the usual drop in the eosinophil count will not occur because the adrenal cortex cannot produce the hormones normally released in response to ACTH stimulation. Because patients with Addison's disease have delayed excretion of water loads, large volumes of water may be given as a diuretic test. The amounts of steroids, especially plasma cortisol, in the serum are decreased.

Treatment. Treatment includes 25 to 50 mg/day doses of cortisone or hydrocortisone. When stress is increased, the daily doses of steroids must be increased. Diets high in sodium (up to 10 gm daily) may be needed.

Secondary chronic adrenocortical deficiency is related most commonly to the administration of steroids over long periods of time for the treatment of other illnesses, such as arthritis or bronchitis. When steroids are administered for an extended period, the adrenal cortex atrophies. Thus when stress is encountered, the adrenals cannot produce enough hormones. For this reason, the steroid dosage must be increased in stress situations.

Nurse's Responsibilities. Upon admission of all patients, determine which are taking steroids; report these to the physician.

Observe for negative effects, such as electrolyte imbalances, of steroid administration.

Observe for responses to stress and for symptoms that show an increased need for hormones (such as symptoms of hypovolemia proceeding to shock).

Assist in regulating a slow withdrawal from steroid drugs.

Observe for and report signs and symptoms that indicate ulcer formation (steroids increase the production of hydrochloric acid).

Perform necessary tasks in skin care.

Observe for symptoms of increasing loss of electrolytes.

Hyperfunction (Cushing's Syndrome)

Hyperfunction, or Cushing's syndrome, is the overproduction of hydrocortisone or other steroids. Cushing's syndrome has two major cause categories. In the first, the cause is found directly in the adrenal glands. Such problems as adenomas and carcinomas of the adrenal glands are examples of direct adrenal malfunction. Hyperplasia of the adrenals, also a direct malfunction, is caused by overactivity of the hypothalamus, which in turn increases ACTH. In the second category, the cause is the overproduction of ACTH despite an increased level of plasma cortisol. In other words, the negative feedback mechanism is not working. This is particularly evident in pituitary adenomas, Cushing's syndrome, or non-endocrine tumors of the ACTH secreting pituitary.

Recognition. The major symptoms of hyperfunction are related to the increased amount of glucocorticoids and mineralcorticoids in the blood. Changes in the skin are frequently seen. Loss of elasticity results in fragility of the blood vessels and the development of purplish streaks on the skin. Patients bruise easily, with purple to black **ecchymoses.** The face is usually flushed and oily. Patients with Cushing's syndrome usually develop excessive body and facial hair (hirsutism) and a thinning of scalp hair. This is caused by an excess of androgens. Another effect of excessive androgens in the female is acne. Table 16-2 lists by body system the basic signs and symptoms of hyperadrenalism.

TABLE 16-2. SIGNS AND SYMPTOMS OF OVERPRODUCTION OF ADRENAL HORMONES

System	Signs and Symptoms
Central nervous	Emotional changes including depression, anxiety, irritability, apathy
Cardiovascular	Hypertension; enlarged heart progressing to congestive heart failure and terminating in an edematous state (sodium retention and potassium loss)
Gastrointestinal	Ulcers due to increased pepsin and hydrochloric acid
Reproductive	Loss of libido; impotence; absence of menses
Musculoskeletal	Heavy trunks, thin extremities, moon face, buffalo hump (kyphosis of the spine), fat pads under cheeks, bulging eye balls, eventual development of stretch streaks on hips and shoulders

Laboratory Tests. The serum hormonal level of steroids is increased. A urinalysis will show increased levels of 17-hydroxycorticoids and 17-ketosteroids.

If, following administration of ACTH, a serum hormonal test indicates increased hormonal production, hyperfunction exists.

Aldosterone levels may be normal or elevated. Androgens are increased; estrogens may also be increased.

Treatment. In some cases, the patient with hyperfunction will undergo spontaneous remission; however, this is rare. If the problem is caused by a tumor, surgery to remove the tumor is indicated. In cases of hyperplasia, a bilateral adrenalectomy may be necessary. The adrenals may be irradiated to decrease the amount of adrenal tissue producing hormones. Suppressive drugs, such as amphenone B, may also be used. There is the possibility that hormone production may drop too low with any of these treatments.

Nurse's Responsibilities. Monitor and report signs and symptoms suggestive of extracellular volume excess (hypertension, edema, breathing difficulty).

Report symptoms suggestive of hyperglycemia (lethargy, nausea, vomiting, diarrhea, polyuria, excessive thirst).

Remove excess oils from skin.

Initiate ulcer prevention measures by the use of drugs or milk products according to physician's directions.

Provide emotional support, recognizing personality changes.

Observe closely for shock after adrenalectomy (the sympathetic nervous system will replace the adrenalin lost by the adrenalectomy).

BIBLIOGRAPHY

Beland, I.: Clinical Nursing: Pathophysiological and Psychosocial Approaches, ed. 2. The Macmillan Company, New York, 1970.

Burrell, Z., and Burrell, L.: Intensive Nursing Care. The C. V. Mosby Company, St. Louis, 1969.

Kupperman, H.: Human Endocrinology. F. A. Davis Company, Philadelphia, 1963.

Moon, H.: The Adrenal Cortex. Harper & Row Publishers, Inc., New York, 1961.

Nichols, T., Nugent, C. A., and Tyler, F. H.: Steroid laboratory test in the diagnosis of Cushing's syndrome. Am. J. Med. 45:116, 1968.

O'Malley, B. W.: Mechanisms of action of steroid hormones. N. Eng. J. Med. 284:370, 1971.

Ravel, R.: Clinical Laboratory Medicine. Year Book Medical Publishers, Inc., Chicago, 1970.

Rosenfeld, M. G. (ed.): Manual of Medical Therapeutics, ed. 2. Little, Brown and Company, Boston, 1971.

Turner, D.: General Endocrinology. W. B. Saunders Company, Philadelphia, 1966.

Williams, R.: Textbook of Endocrinology. W. B. Saunders Company, Philadelphia, 1962.

NOTES

17

Congestive Heart Failure

Because the entire body is dependent on adequate circulation for distribution of nutrients and elimination of waste products, any decrease in the pumping action which circulates the blood will produce many contingent problems. For this reason congestive heart failure is closely related to fluid, electrolyte, and renal problems.

Pathophysiology

In congestive heart failure, the heart is unable to pump with sufficient force to perfuse the body's tissues in proportion to their requirements. For proper metabolism, the heart must pump adequate oxygen and nutrients to all body tissues via the systemic circulation. Oxygen is especially needed to metabolize glucose and fats to carbon dioxide and water. The stage at which the heart is no longer able to function adequately is called compensatory decompensation.

Congestive heart failure is associated with three causative factors: inadequate ventricular filling, increased work load of the heart muscles, and deterioration of the myocardium due to a decreased blood supply.

Inadequate ventricular filling is due to obstructions, such as in mitral stenosis secondary to rheumatic heart disease. In this disease process, inflammation eventually causes scarring and stenosing of the opening.

Another possible cause of inadequate ventricular filling is a pressure build-up outside of the ventricles, decreasing the area in which the ventricles can expand. This type of extracardiac pressure can be found in dysfunctions such as chronic **pericarditis** or cardiac **tamponade** in which excessive fluids gather around the heart.

A third cause of inadequate filling is arrhythmias. An example is tachycardia, in which the increased heart rate does not allow sufficient time for the ventricle to fill adequately, thereby decreasing cardiac output. Cardiac output, which is the amount of blood pumped with each beat, is equal to the heart rate times the stroke volume. With a pulse rate of 70, average cardiac output is 4 liters per minute. Increased cardiac output is achieved with a more effective pump, improved venous return, and a normal pulse rate. An increased rate will increase output up to the point where the ventricles do not have sufficient time to fill.

The second major causative factor of congestive heart failure, an increased

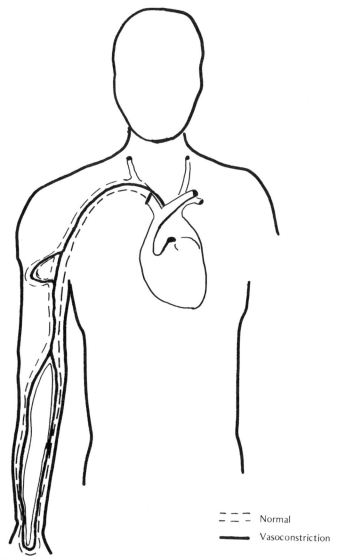

Normal

Vasoconstriction

Figure 17-1.   Vasoconstriction. The broken line indicates a normal vascular bed. The solid line shows the reduction of the vascular bed due to vasoconstriction.

work load for the heart muscles, may be due to increased resistance to the peripheral vascular system because of narrowed vessels, as shown in Figure 17-1. With vasoconstriction the heart must pump harder to overcome the increased resistance. In hypertension, the peripheral vessels may have become narrowed due to arteriosclerosis (hardening of the arteries), thereby heightening the peripheral resistance. Peripheral hypertension specifically magnifies the work of the left heart. Pulmonary hypertension makes it harder for the right heart to pump blood into the lungs via the pulmonary artery. Pulmonary hypertension may be increased by pulmonary or vascular diseases.

Another cause of an increased work load for the heart is anemia. The lack of red blood cells and the resulting lack of hemoglobin decreases the amount of oxygen carried to the cells; therefore the heart must work harder to circulate the blood more rapidly. Any disease that increases the body's need for oxygen and nutrients will heighten the work of the heart.

Decreased amounts of fluid in the body also cause the heart to work harder and faster to carry oxygen and nutrients to the cells by increasing the rate of circulation. If the patient has a failing heart, this added strain aggravates the failure.

The third causative factor of heart failure is a deterioration of the myocardium due to a decreased functional blood supply. The heart, like every other muscle in the body, must receive oxygen in order to perform its task. An inadequate blood supply will cause failure of its pumping action. An inadequate blood supply may be due to coronary ischemia secondary to plugging of the coronary vessels from fatty plaques or clots with consequent death of tissue (myocardial **infarction**). Tissue death results in inadequate myocardial pump action because the "dead" or scarred muscles have lost their contractibility. This can create a circular compounding problem, because the irregular beats and rhythms will also lessen the normal filling time of the ventricles, further decreasing the cardiac output, thereby lessening even more the amount of blood going to the coronary vessels. Muscles in an anaerobic cycle produce lactic acid, inducing metabolic acidosis. In other words, metabolic acidosis is due to inadequate tissue perfusion.

Chronic Congestive Heart Failure. Heart failure can be either chronic or acute. Chronic heart failure occurs when injury or decompensation takes place slowly. The symptoms develop over a period of days, weeks, or months. The cardinal signs are fluid congestion in the peripheral tissues and anoxia caused by the diminished blood flow to the tissues resulting from the pump failure. The most common early symptoms are dyspnea and fatigue.

Chronic congestive heart failure may involve the right, the left, or both sides of the heart. The most common etiologies are hypertension and arteriosclerosis, although there are numerous other possible causes.

Acute Heart Failure. In acute heart failure, there is a sudden loss of effective cardiac contractions, and thus a reduced cardiac output. Acute heart failure results in an engorgement of the lungs causing acute pulmonary edema. When fluid enters the lungs, the situation becomes a medical emergency.

Mechanisms of Cardiac Failure

The mechanisms of cardiac failure are very complex and at this time are not completely understood. There are two basic theoretical models: the forward theory and the backward theory. The forward theory describes a condition in which the heart cannot pump out the amount of blood needed by the peripheral vascular system. There is a decrease in cardiac output, progressing into the low output syndrome seen in cardiogenic shock. Low cardiac output results in ischemia in all periphery. Since one-fourth of the cardiac output perfuses the kidneys, even the kidneys are affected, producing a low renal output.

The backward theory describes a situation in which the heart is receiving more blood than it can pump out. The blood therefore backs away from the heart like water behind a dam. The blood can be trapped at two places. The right heart can dam the blood back to the liver, neck veins, and extremities; and the left heart can dam the blood back to the lungs.

Congestive heart failure is usually a combination of both forward and backward mechanisms.

Right Heart Failure. Right heart failure is usually a backward failure causing systemic venous congestion.

Left Heart Failure. Left heart failure is predominately a backward failure with the blood damming back into the lungs, causing acute pulmonary edema. The extra blood in the pulmonary capillaries may escape into the alveoli causing the patient to "drown" in his own fluids. Fluid in the main bronchi causes congestion and produces mucus and a productive cough, possibly blood-tinged. The rupture of distended capillaries produces blood-tinged mucus causing the **hemoptysis.** Moist **rales** or **rhonchi** can be heard as air flows through the fluid in the alveoli. Dyspnea is an action initiated by the dilated pulmonary vessels. The reduced size of the respiratory air sacs causes inadequate oxygenation of the blood, further aggravating the problem.

Compensatory Mechanisms

In congestive heart failure, all the organs of the body endeavor to counteract the effects of the failing pump. It is interesting to note that some of the compensatory mechanisms become self-defeating. Figure 17-2 illustrates these self-defeating effects.

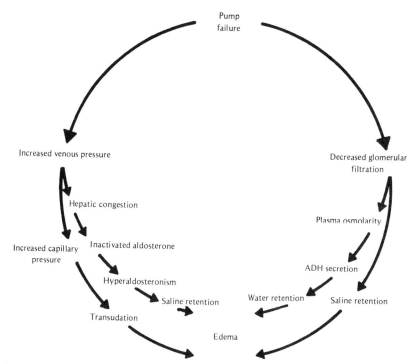

Figure 17-2. Schematic representation of the self-defeating effects of the compensatory mechanisms.

Cardiac Response

During congestive heart failure, the decreased pumping action leads to incomplete emptying of the ventricles; therefore less blood circulates through the lungs and less oxygenation takes place. The incomplete evacuation and decreased arterial blood volume cause *increased venous*-blood volume leading to pulmonary edema. While the inadequate emptying of the left heart is producing pulmonary edema, the back pressure of the right heart is causing systemic edema. Pulmonary edema may be recognized by signs of anoxia, such as paroxysmal nocturnal dyspnea (PND) and orthopnea, and also by early signs of anoxia to the brain and heart. Systemic edema can be recognized by engorged neck veins, liver congestion, and by pedal and presacral edema. Edema in the periphery and abdomen is due to an elevated hydrostatic pressure in the veins secondary to the increased venous blood volume. The elevated hydrostatic pressure pushes the fluid out of the veins into the interstitial spaces. The cardiac compensatory response is to increase output by increasing the rate of contraction of the heart muscle. This is ultimately a self-defeating reaction, since extremely rapid heart contractions do not allow sufficient time for the ventricles to fill adequately.

Adrenocortical Response

The anterior pituitary interprets decreased arterial blood pressure as a stress situation. The body cells indicate a need for more fluid (saline) to increase the arterial blood supply to the head. Through the negative feedback mechanism and corticotropin releasing factor **(CRF)**, the anterior pituitary is stimulated to release adrenocorticotrophic hormone (ACTH) which in turn causes the adrenal cortex to secrete the steroids, glucocorticoids and mineralcorticoids. The mineralcorticoids, especially, cause the retention of sodium and chloride and thus water. The retention of extracellular fluid actually compounds congestive heart failure by increasing the already excessive blood volume. It also adds all the problems inherent in an extracellular fluid excess.

An additional complication caused by the retention of sodium and chloride may be the loss of potassium through the urine.

Neural Response

The neural response, like the adrenocortical response, is triggered by the lowered arterial blood pressure. The lowered arterial blood pressure decreases the perfusion of the brain, stimulating the posterior pituitary to release ADH. ADH causes the distal tubules of the kidney to retain water in an attempt to increase the arterial blood pressure. This compensatory response is also self-defeating because it increases the burden on the failing heart.

Renal Response

Decreased cardiac output and peripheral vasoconstriction decrease renal perfusion. In response to the stress hormones (glucocorticoids and mineralcorticoids), the kidney tubules retain sodium, chloride, and water, as shown in Figure 17-3. The kidneys also release renin, a parahormone, to raise the blood pressure. Erythropoietin, another parahormone of the kidneys, may be secreted in the stress response to increase the release of red blood cells to carry more oxygen to the peripheral tissues.

Hepatic Response

The damming up of the venous blood flow as a result of peripheral vasoconstriction increases the amount of blood in the liver and causes congestion. Liver congestion accompanies right heart failure. Normally, the liver

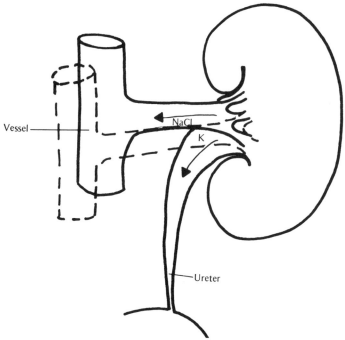

Figure 17-3. Schematic representation of electrolyte movement. Due to a stress response sodium and chloride are reabsorbed into the bloodstream while potassium is excreted.

breaks down excess hormones (steroids, ADH); however, with congestion, this function fails and the excessive hormones cause the undesirable effects already listed in the adrenal and renal responses.

Peripheral Vascular Response

The decreased cardiac output and arterial blood pressure eventually progress to cardiogenic shock. The sympathetic nervous system initiates the stress response by releasing adrenalin and noradrenalin, causing vasoconstriction of all major peripheral vessels except the coronary vessels. Vasoconstriction decreases the amount of oxygen available to the body cells to carry on metabolism (anaerobic metabolism). Without oxygen, the carbohydrates are catabolized only to the lactic acid stage and lactic acidosis results. Vasoconstriction increases arterial resistance and forces the heart to pump harder, thus aggravating the pump failure. Vasoconstriction also causes increased venous return to the heart, adding to the already existing overload. Again, this mechanism is actually self-defeating.

A further complication of the peripheral vascular response is caused by the increased adrenalin, which, in addition to stimulating vasoconstriction, also directly stimulates the heart. Because the heart cannot respond to this stimulus with effective beats, the increased adrenalin may result in further arrhythmias.

Respiratory Response

The compensatory action of the respiratory system responds to two stimuli: adrenalin in the blood and lactic acidosis. Adrenalin, which is produced by the sympathetic nervous system and the adrenal medulla, causes the bronchioles of the lungs to dilate and increases the rate of breathing. In lactic acidosis, which is the result of an inadequate amount of oxygen to metabolize glucose, the bronchioles dilate and the rate of breathing increases in an attempt to increase the amount of available oxygen to alleviate the lactic acidosis and to convert glucose into the energy so desperately needed by the body. In pulmonary edema fluid is extravasated into the interstitial spaces in the lungs causing rales and rhonchi.

Deviations in Fluid, Electrolyte, and Acid-Base Balance

Extracellular Fluid Excess

There are several factors which combine to create the extracellular fluid excess found in congestive heart failure. As the pump fails, renal perfusion is decreased causing the kidney tubules to retain sodium, chloride, and water. The stimulated stress response results in the production of steroids (especially mineralcorticoids) which also cause saline retention.

Right heart failure, which frequently causes backward pressure, further aggravates the situation by increasing the venous blood pressure. As venous pressure builds up, it elevates the hydrostatic pressure in the plasma which pushes blood into the interstitial spaces.

These combined factors of extracellular fluid excess can lead to abdominal distention from liver congestion (right heart failure) and pulmonary edema (left heart failure). The hematocrit and hemoglobin are reduced due to the extracellular fluid excess.

Hypokalemia

Hypokalemia, like extracellular fluid excess, is caused by several interrelated factors. When the kidneys respond to the steroids, stimulated by the stress mechanism, they retain sodium and chloride and excrete potassium. Vomiting and diarrhea, which also accompany the stress response, further deplete the body's potassium. A potassium deficit is compounded by the administration of potent diuretics and digitalis preparations. The deficit can become so acute that it results in digitalis intoxication.

A potassium deficit may exist as a result of the conditions listed above, and yet the potassium reading may be elevated because of the presence of lactic acidosis. However, as the acidosis is corrected, theoretically hydrogen ions move out of the cell and potassium ions move back into the cell, magnifying the extracellular potassium deficit.

If congestive heart failure becomes more severe and oliguria develops, the potassium level will increase to hyperkalemia.

Intracellular Fluid Excess

The stress reponse elicited by decreased arterial pressure causes the pituitary to secrete ADH to retain water. The serum sodium reading is low because of the water excess.

Metabolic Lactic Acidosis

The chain of events in this imbalance is that the decreased cardiac output causes decreased renal perfusion, resulting in the retention of nitrogenous waste products which increase the retention of hydrogen ions. Hypoxia causes anaerobic metabolism of carbohydrates which increases the production of lactic acid, resulting in metabolic lactic acidosis. However, metabolic acidosis is more frequently seen with a cardiopulmonary arrest.

Recognition

It is more important for the nurse to recognize the degree and the rate of congestive heart failure than to be able to distinguish which side of the heart is failing. Table 17-1 gives signs and symptoms elicited by altered function.

TABLE 17-1. SIGNS AND SYMPTOMS INDICATIVE OF ALTERED FUNCTIONS

Signs and Symptoms	Altered Function
Dyspnea, **SOB** with or without exertion, paroxysmal nocturnal dyspnea, orthopnea, Cheyne-Stokes respiration	Pulmonary congestion with fluid from left-sided failure; pulmonary capillary pressure increases, lessening available space to diffuse gases, leading to hypoxemia, hypercapnia, and hemoptysis; increased pulmonary capillary pressure pushes blood into alveoli leading to foamy, blood-tinged sputum; increased pulmonary congestion heightens work of right heart leading to failure
Apprehension, irritability, restlessness, sensorium decreased to stupor, coma, cough reflex	Dyspnea leads to less oxygen to central nervous system; nerve tissue unable to function without oxygen and nutrients; increased fluid in lungs stimulates cough reflex
Systemic edema, pitting edema, liver congestion, ascites, sacral edema when recumbent, neck vein distention, increased central venous pressure	Retention of fluid in interstitial spaces secondary to increased hydrostatic pressure in capillaries resulting from increased venous pressure due to retention of saline; capillary pressure high and tissue pressure low in veins draining upper and lower parts of body
Anorexia, nausea, vomiting, diarrhea or constipation	Decreased blood flow to GI system in *stress* response; vagal reflexes initiated by cardiac changes also stimulate GI nerves; reflex vomiting possibly due to hypoxia of brain tissue; may be decreased or increased peristalsis in stress
Fever, diaphoresis	Sympathetic nervous system *(stress* response) stimulated to increase heart rate to augment cardiac output; speeds metabolism
Palpitation, tachycardia, gallop rhythm, pulsus alternans	Change in heart rhythm related to hypoxia of the myocardium
Oliguria	Decreased cardiac output leads to inadequate renal perfusion; retention of nitrogenous waste products and hydrogen ions results in acidosis

Laboratory tests of cardiac, renal, and hepatic functions are needed to evaluate a patient with congestive heart failure. Analyzed together, these test results, listed in Table 17-2, indicate the degree or confirm the presence of congestive heart failure or related heart problems.

TABLE 17-2. LABORATORY TEST RESULTS BY FUNCTION

Function	Laboratory Results
Cardiac	Evaluate electrical impulses (EKG) for arrhythmias; Xray for size and position of heart and great vessels; cardiac output decreased; circulatory time increased (arm to tongue test in left heart failure); (arm to lung test in right heart failure); venous pressure increased (CVP normal = 6-12 cm of water); CPK↑ with damage to the myocardium
Renal	BUN increased with prerenal failure or renal failure from decreased perfusion; creatinine increases after BUN; urine osmolarity increased; high specific gravity; serum osmolarity decreased; proteinuria; serum Na decreased (ICF excess); serum hemoglobin and hematocrit decreased (ECF excess)
Hepatic	SGOT, SGPT, lactic dehydrogenase (LDH), and alkaline phosphatase increased due to decreased liver flow; liver hypoxia; slight increase of bilirubin; hypoxia results in failure to synthesize albumin, increasing the edematous state because of decreasing colloid osmotic pressure in blood; some prolongation of prothrombin time due to failure to synthesize; hypoglycemia; inadequate storage of glycogen in liver and increased catabolism of glucose to lactic acid with hypoxia; serum CO_2 decreased, pH decreased with lactic metabolic acidosis

Treatment

The major goals in the treatment of cardiac failure are to increase the contractility of the heart muscles (the pump action) and to decrease the peripheral demands upon the heart for oxygen and nutrients until the pump action is restored. Cardiotonics are the most frequently used means of improving the pump action; rest and limited activity during the acute phase decrease the work load of the heart. Aminophylline decreases bronchospasms and increases the output of the heart. Morphine lessens anxiety and pain while decreasing dyspnea. Oxygen may or may not be used. Diuretics are used to decrease the amount of fluid circulating through the heart. Anticoagulants may be used to decrease clot formation. Rotating tourniquets may be used to reduce the volume load on the heart.

The diet is usually low in sodium (250 mg to 1000 mg) and includes fluid restriction to lessen the work load of the heart. Cardiac arrhythmias must be monitored and treated.

If cardiogenic shock ensues, primarily after a myocardial infarction, treatment may be the use of vasopressors. Forward failure, which is cardiogenic shock, is the least well understood of the shock syndromes. This type of shock results in inadequate tissue perfusion. The mortality rate, even with treatment, is 80 per cent or more. Pacing may be required if a bradycardia or heart block develops with the hypoxia.

To summarize, the primary treatment for congestive heart failure consists of the three Ds: digitalis, diuretics, and diet.

Table 17-3 is meant to clarify the goal of each nursing task and to em-
phasize the reason for their implementation.

TABLE 17-3. NURSE RESPONSIBILITIES AND THEIR RATIONALE

Responsibility	*Rationale*
Monitor cardiac patterns	Identifies rhythm changes secondary to hypoxia
Start "keep open" (**KVO**) intravenous fluid according to institutional policy*	May be needed for emergency drugs
Administer oxygen as directed	Lessens hypoxia and metabolic lactic acidosis
Provide emotional support	Decreases tension thus decreases oxygen need; avoids vicious cycle of tension and hypoxia
Observe and record vital signs and report changes	Indicate fluid overload; cardiogenic shock; arrhythmias
Some sources do not recommend taking temperatures rectally even if oxygen is being administered; axillary temperature may be acceptable.	Thermometer may stimulate the vagus in the rectal sphincter causing or aggravating arrhythmias.
Have emergency drugs readily available according to *institutional policy*	Administer drugs for crisis
Lidocaine bolus and/or drip Atropine Sodium bicarbonate	Used commonly for arrhythmias Used commonly for bradycardia Used commonly for metabolic acidosis due to cardiac arrest
Administer drugs as ordered; observe for side effects of diuretics and digitalis (indirect diuretic)	Diuretics may cause potassium deficit
Elevate head of bed slightly unless patient is in shock	Decreases venous return; lowers abdominal pressure; increases lung space, i.e., ventilation; facilitates respiration
Suction orally as needed	Clears airway to aid ventilation and prevent hypoxia
Note and chart the appearance of skin for moistness, dryness, coolness	Changes may indicate further stress response
Observe for signs of increased edema; obtain daily weight	Increases may be indicative of further saline retention
Chart fluid intake and output	Assesses adequate perfusion of kidneys
Restrict fluids as ordered	Decreases fluid volume
Restrict sodium in diet as ordered	Decreases fluid volume caused by saline excess

TABLE 17-3. (continued)

Assure rest according to the physician's orders. Guidelines (unless specified otherwise): Do *not* allow patient to pull self up in bed, strain on bedpan or commode, cross legs, or massage limbs	Lessens the work load and the burning of nutrients in decreased oxygenated state
Do actively move the patients arms and legs gently several times daily and assist patient to turn	Maintains muscle strength; discourages formation of peripheral emboli
Rotate tourniquets	Helps relieve skin breakdown secondary to anoxia
Initiate rehabilitative teaching relative to circumstances	Assists patient and family to cope with change in body image and/or life style
Identify possible social agency referrals pertinent to patient/family	Utilizes agencies that have services available to aid the patient and family in time of need

*These are suggested procedures that vary with the institution; standing orders are recommended.

The treatment plan must be followed closely and adapted as necessary. It is especially crucial to note subtle changes in edema, respiration, consciousness, apprehension, urine output, and circulatory status. Complications such as peripheral emboli must be prevented. The major treatment objectives for the patient with congestive heart failure are always to reduce the work load of the heart and to increase circulation to the periphery in order to keep the body properly oxygenated.

BIBLIOGRAPHY

Beland, I.: Clinical Nursing: Pathophysiological and Psychological Approaches, ed. 2. The Macmillan Company, New York, 1970.

Boric, E.: Intensive care of a cardiac patient. Am. J. Nurs. 65:131, 1965.

Brunner, L., et al.: Textbook of Medical-Surgical Nursing, ed. 3. J. B. Lippincott Company, Philadelphia, 1975.

Burrell, Z. L., Jr., and Burrell, L. O.: Intensive Nursing Care. The C. V. Mosby Company, St. Louis, 1969.

Clark, N. F.: Pump failure. Nurs. Clin. North Am. 7:529, 1972.

Dean, V.: Measuring venous blood pressure. Am. J. Nurs. 63:70, 1963.

Guyton, A. C.: Textbook of Medical Physiology, ed. 5. W. B. Saunders Company, Philadelphia, 1976.

Hazeltine, L. S.: The weeks of healing. Am. J. Nurs. 64:14, 1964.

The Heart of the Home. American Heart Association, New York.

Hurst, J. W., and Logne, R. B.: The Heart, ed. 2. McGraw-Hill, New York, 1970.

Rosenfeld, M. G. (ed.): Manual of Medical Therapeutics, ed. 2. Little, Brown and Company, Boston, 1971.

Scribner, B. H., and Burnell, J. M.: Teaching Syllabus for the Course on Fluid and Electrolyte Balance, ed. 7. University of Washington, Seattle, 1969.

Shabetai, R.: Symposium: Pericardial disease. Am. J. Cardiol. 26:445, 1970.

The sympathetic nervous system in heart failure. Hosp. Practice 5:31, 1970.

Wintrobe, M. M., et al. (eds.): Harrison's Principles of Internal Medicine, ed. 6. McGraw-Hill, New York, 1970.

NOTES

162

NOTES

18

Shock

The quality of care for patients in shock is largely dependent upon the nurse's informed observation and ability to correctly interpret her observations. Observation alone is only the recognition of a condition or a behavior. The nurse must also be able to produce coherence and order from the jumble of her observations in order to correctly interpret them. Acute observations, sound judgments, and proper actions are proportionate to the nurse's knowledge and understanding of and experience with the subject.

This chapter contains information and discusses situations to help the nurse anticipate conditions prior to their occurrence in the potential shock victim. This chapter also stresses specific actions that the nurse may take independently, as well as actions which will assist the doctor in his treatment plan.

Definition and Classification of Shock

Shock may be due to physical or psychological causes. However, both result in a discrepancy between the circulating blood volume and the size of the vascular bed. Figure 18-1 illustrates this effect. The primary definition for shock, regardless of type, is "an abnormal physiological state characterized by a disproportion between the circulating blood volume and the size of the vascular bed resulting in circulatory failure and tissue anoxia."[*]

Numerous etiologies for the shock state have been identified. However, as Figure 18-2 shows, shock can be regarded as the result of three abnormal events: any fluid volume loss (hypovolemic shock), cardiac pump failure (cardiogenic shock), and loss of peripheral vascular tone or vasodilation (neurogenic shock). Bordicks includes a fourth type called vasogenic shock[+] which is also due to vasodilation, but is related to the direct action of toxic substances on the blood vessels. The term hematogenic shock may also be used. This term refers to the loss of plasma and cellular particles, i.e., whole blood, and thus is a type of hypovolemic shock. Shock may be due to one or any combination of these three pathophysiological events.

---

[*]Kathleen J. Bordicks: Patterns of Shock, The Macmillan Co., New York, 1965, p. 4.
[+]Ibid.

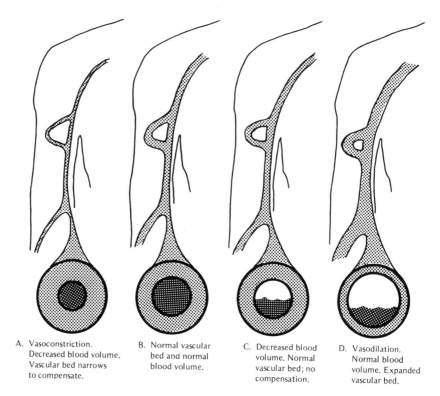

A. Vasoconstriction.
Decreased blood volume.
Vascular bed narrows
to compensate.

B. Normal vascular
bed and normal
blood volume.

C. Decreased blood
volume. Normal
vascular bed; no
compensation.

D. Vasodilation.
Normal blood
volume. Expanded
vascular bed.

Figure 18-1. Discrepancy between amount of blood volume and size of circulating bed.

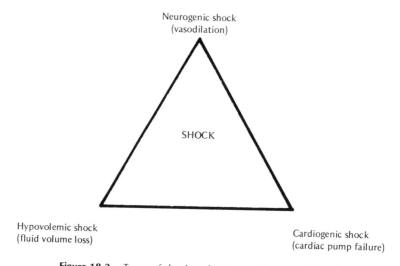

Neurogenic shock
(vasodilation)

SHOCK

Hypovolemic shock
(fluid volume loss)

Cardiogenic shock
(cardiac pump failure)

Figure 18-2. Types of shock and corresponding altered function.

Although classification into these three basic types is an oversimplification of the complex state of shock, it is a useful guide when observing persons susceptible to a specific type of shock. It will also aid in instituting proper care under the physician's guidance.

Each of the factors—blood volume, cardiac output, and vascular tone— can be altered considerably without resulting in inadequate tissue perfusion as long as the compensatory mechanisms of the body are functioning properly.

Physiology Review

As already indicated, the body depends on three main factors to maintain the correct proportion of blood to the size of the vascular bed: blood volume, cardiac output, and vascular tone. A significant variation in any of these three hemodynamic factors may result in shock.

The average-sized man (75 kg) has a total blood volume of 4.5 to 5.5 liters. Plasma is approximately 90 per cent water and 10 per cent solutes which are either crystalloid or colloid. The solutes may also be classified according to their ionizing ability as electrolytes or non-electrolytes (see Section II). When the volume of plasma changes, the type of filtrate reaching the cells for tissue metabolism also changes. Blood plasma, however, is only one of the body's three fluids. The others are the interstitial fluid and the intracellular fluid. Figure 18-3 shows the distribution of the fluids in the body. A loss of any of the body's fluids may precipitate shock, because they all ultimately affect the volume of blood circulating through the body.

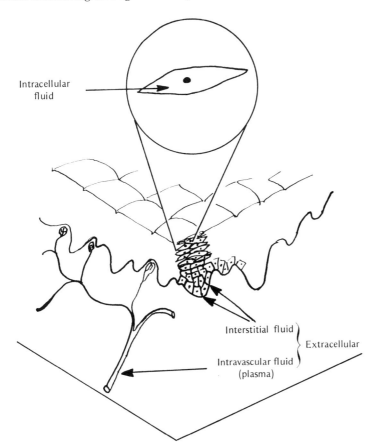

Intracellular fluid

Interstitial fluid ⎫
                    ⎬ Extracellular
Intravascular fluid ⎭
(plasma)

Figure 18-3.   Fluid distribution.

The primary function of the circulatory system is transportation. The cells will not receive sufficient oxygen and nutrients if the blood volume is inadequate. The result of this deficiency is cellular hypoxia.

Pathophysiology

The pathophysiology of shock involves a dynamic interchange between blood volume, cardiac output, and the amount of peripheral vascular resistance or tone. If the quantity of blood does not change, the amount of blood that circulates to the tissues results from an interaction between cardiac output and peripheral tone. The term "peripheral tone" includes both vasoconstriction and vasodilation. Blood pressure is determined by the force with which the heart is pushing the blood (indicated by the systolic reading) and the resistance or back pressure the heart meets (indicated by the diastolic reading). The resistance of the vessels is largely determined by their size. The more the vessels are constricted, the higher the resistance and the harder the heart must pump to circulate the blood through the vessels. Thus shock is not merely defined as a low blood pressure. In fact, the blood pressure can remain unchanged while the amount of the blood circulating to the tissues varies. Figure 18-4 demonstrates a comparison of these three factors. As the figure illustrates, the amount of urinary output is a more reliable guide to tissue perfusion than is blood pressure.

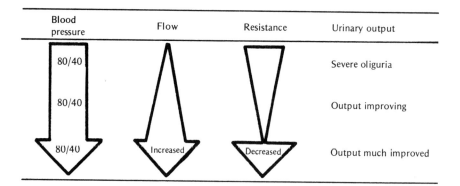

Blood pressure	Flow	Resistance	Urinary output
80/40			Severe oliguria
80/40			Output improving
80/40	Increased	Decreased	Output much improved

Figure 18-4. Hemodynamics in shock. Although blood pressure remains constant, as the cardiac output is increased and the peripheral vascular resistance is decreased, kidney perfusion and urinary output improves. This indicates an improved total body tissue perfusion.

The patient will exhibit identifiable signs and symptoms because of the decreased amount of blood reaching the vital organs. The central nervous system and the cardiovascular system react early to this stress. Characteristic manifestations seen clinically include pallor, cold and moist skin, collapsed peripheral veins, sluggishly filling capillaries, rapid "thready" pulse proceeding to irregular pulse, decreased urinary output, changes in mental state or sensorium, and a fall in blood pressure. Lactic acidosis may be associated with this state because oxygen is inadequate to metabolize carbohydrates. A primary indication of adequacy of tissue perfusion is urinary output. A decreased urinary output usually indicates inadequate tissue perfusion. This list of signs and symptoms illustrates the fact that shock is not merely the lowering of the blood pressure.

Hypovolemic Shock

Hemorrhage and gastrointestinal bleeding are typical causes of hypovolemic shock, but fluid loss from vomiting, diarrhea, burns, peritonitis, and trauma are also common causes. Hypovolemic shock can be due to hemorrhage involving the loss of whole blood or the loss of only the plasma portion of the blood, the latter resulting in **hemoconcentration.**

Hemorrhage. Shock due to hemorrhage relates to the decreased volume of circulating blood. Hemorrhage is the loss of blood from the bloodstream due to a disruption in the continuity of one or more blood vessels (arterial, venous, or capillary). Possible causes include physical or chemical injury to the body. More specific examples are the rupture of or injury to a blood vessel from the slipping of a suture, erosion of a vessel by drainage tubes, tumor or infection, interference with the clotting mechanism as in hemophilia, or fragile capillaries as in vitamin C deficiency. Bleeding may also occur from a body orifice, such as gastrointestinal bleeding, or from an incision site. It may collect under subcutaneous tissue as hematoma, or in a body cavity.

Hemorrhage may be classified as gradual or sudden, internal or external, and by type of vessel. The types of vascular bleeding are further categorized as arterial (bright red and spurting), venous (dark red and continuous) and capillary (either bright red or dark red and oozing). Gradual, internal, and capillary bleeding are the most difficult to detect by early shock symptoms.

Body's Response to Hemorrhage. When a patient has lost over 500 cc of whole blood (for an average weight of 75 kg), the effect of this loss becomes evident from certain specific body changes. All of these effects of blood loss reinforce the hypoxia and further increase tissue damage. The decreased capacity of the body to deliver sufficient blood and oxygen to the cells is related to the decreased volume and the decreased number of red blood cells.

Part of the problem in hypoxia is that the body's defense mechanisms automatically eliminate general tissue perfusion and instead concentrate on keeping the blood flow steady to the more vital organs.

A decreased blood volume excites three initial responses. The first, vasoconstriction, lessens the size of the vascular bed in order to maintain systemic blood pressure. This change can be indicated by a slight rising of the diastolic pressure in early shock. The second, the constriction of arterioles, increases peripheral resistance to help maintain systemic blood pressure. The third, the transfer of fluid from the interstitial fluid to the blood, is stimulated by the adrenocortical hormones. This transfer of fluid increases the blood volume, again with the objective of increasing the systemic blood pressure.

The body tries to control local bleeding in several ways. A reflex contraction (vascular spasm) of the blood vessel occurs. This is a function of the lumen of the vessel based on the physical principle that the smaller the opening, the less blood can be evacuated. The muscles also contract to aid in reducing the size of the lumen of the vessel. Muscle contraction further aids the body by immobilizing the injured part. The inside layer of the vessel curls inward to increase occlusion of the vessel.

A clot begins its formation in the terminal portion of the vessel. The traumatized tissue releases tissue **thromboplastin** (thrombokinase). Platelets adhere to the broken edges of the blood vessels. As the platelets rupture, they release plasma thromboplastin. Calcium, globulin, and several plasma proteins are necessary in activating the thromboplastins. Thromboplastins, calcium, and globulin then act as catalysts to convert prothrombin, a plasma protein produced by the liver, to thrombin. Vitamin K is necessary for the production of prothrombin.

Another plasma protein produced by the liver is fibrinogen. The thrombin produced through the combined actions of thromboplastins, calcium, globulin, and prothrombin, acts as a catalyst in converting fibrinogen to fibrin. The fibrin then builds a mesh of threads to trap red blood cells, white blood cells, and platelets to form a clot. Serum, which is actually plasma minus the fibrinogen, will collect around the clot.

The clot will be retracted by the fibrin threads, which are attached to the damaged surfaces, contracting and pulling the blood vessel edges together. There must be an adequate number of platelets for a clot to retract successfully, since the platelets form a center for the development of more fibrin threads.

At this point, hopefully, the bleeding is stopped. The clot then organizes to repair the vessel by means of an ingrowth of fibrous cells to form connective tissues, as shown in Figure 18-5. Endothelial cells grow over the vascular surface of the clot to form a new lining. This entire process is a sequential, chain reaction type of mechanism in which the failure of any of the stages results in continuing hemorrhage.

The signs and symptoms of hemorrhage vary according to the site of bleeding and the corresponding amount of blood lost. If blood is trapped in a small cavity such as the cranial or spinal cavity, the symptoms will appear sooner than when the blood is lost to the exterior or a larger cavity. The warning signs and symptoms of cranial or spinal hemorrhage are the same as those of increased intracranial pressure due to a tumor: headache, vertigo, loss of consciousness, convulsions, slower respiration and pulse, vomiting, widening pulse pressure, and unequal pupillary reaction to light. The pulse and respiration rates decrease only in cranial and spinal hemorrhage because of pressure on the cardiac and respiratory control centers.

Signs of blood escaping without pressure within a cavity are largely related to hypovolemia and hypoxia. These signs are reduced blood pressure (reduced volume), nausea and vomiting (stress response), increased pulse and respiration rates (result of stimulation of stress mechanisms), and reduced body temperature (with vasoconstriction). Other signs and symptoms include: apprehension, restlessness, and extreme weakness progressing to unconsciousness; thirst; paleness progressing to pallor and eventually cyanosis (a late sign) of the lips, conjunctiva, and skin; spots before the eyes; ringing in the ears.

Other Types of Hypovolemic Shock. There are four other types of hypovolemic shock in addition to hemorrhage. Burns, with the loss of plasma and electrolytes from the blood to the damaged site, are one type. The edema resulting from the burn creates a third space fluid which cannot be used to maintain systemic circulation.

Diabetic shock (ketoacidosis), the second type of hypovolemic shock, involves a loss of fluid and electrolytes from both body fluid compartments. Much of this fluid loss is caused by hyperglycemia. The

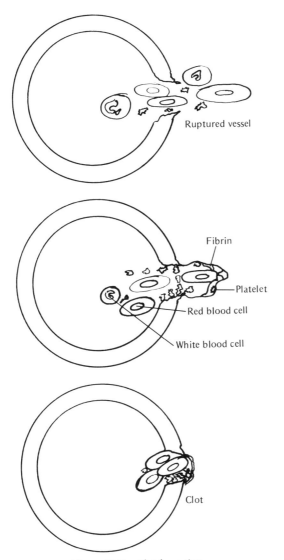

Figure 18-5.   Clot formation.

increased blood sugar acts as an osmotic diuretic, producing a great deal of fluid loss through the urine (polyuria).

A third type of hypovolemic shock involves fluid and electrolyte losses accompanying severe gastrointestinal losses or specific diseases, such as Addison's disease.

The fourth type is due to fluid and electrolyte losses which may follow surgery or its complication.

All types of hypovolemic shock have one important thing in common: loss of fluid volume.

Cardiogenic Shock

The altered function in cardiogenic shock is the failure of the heart to pump enough blood into the systemic circulation to maintain adequate tissue perfusion. This inability of the heart may be due to congestive heart failure (pump failure) or irregular, fast beating which does not allow enough time for the ventricle to fill or have enough strength to pump adequately (atrial flutter, tachycardia, fibrillation). A myocardial infarction may also have lessened the amount of healthy muscular tissue needed for adequate contraction. This is a normovolemic type of shock. A patient with this condition needs the pump failure corrected, rather than fluid replacement.

Neurogenic Shock

Neurogenic shock is due to peripheral vascular dilation. There is no reduction in blood volume, but rather a relocation of a large proportion of blood. The increased size of the vascular bed may be due to nerve stimulation or a nerve block. Simple fainting from severe psychic stimulation is an example of neurogenic shock. The peripheral blood vessels dilate, resulting in a pooling of the blood in the periphery. This shunts blood away from the brain and the person faints. Blood moves back into systemic circulation by the force of gravity, thereby correcting itself.

Other causative factors of neurogenic shock include spinal anesthesia shock, insulin shock (insufficient glucose to brain cells for effective nervous system functioning), postural hypotension, drugs (such as thorazine), and deep general anesthesia (depressing the vasomotor center in the medulla).

Vasogenic Shock

Another type of shock due to peripheral dilatation is vasogenic shock. In this type of shock, a gross peripheral vasodilation is caused by a direct action on the blood vessels. For example, in anaphylactic shock, a foreign protein enters the body and initiates the antigen-antibody response, resulting in the release of histamine. Histamine is a strong peripheral vasodilator and bronchial constrictor. In response to its action, blood is shunted from systemic circulation into the periphery. Once the blood is in the periphery, symptoms of *hypovolemic* shock follow. However, this is *not* hypovolemic shock; it is, rather, normovolemic shock. Administration of large amounts of fluid is not only unnecessary; it is also dangerous. Administration of adrenalin will cause peripheral vasoconstriction and bronchodilation. Antihistaminic drugs (benadryl) may also be given to lessen the antigen-antibody reaction.

Toxic or bacteremic shock is another type of vasogenic shock. Bacteria release toxins that can act directly on the vessels to cause vasodilation. Gram positive organisms release an exotoxin; gram negative organisms release an endotoxin. Gram negative shock is usually more profound and difficult to treat than gram positive shock. Antibiotics are an important part of the treatment.

Stages of Shock   The stages of shock discussed here begin with the onset of shock and end with severe shock. Although these are presented as separate stages, they are, in fact, a continuum with the point of reversibility varying according to the circumstances of each individual case. The role of the nurse is vital. Recognizing changes in the patient that indicate an improving or worsening state and relaying this information to the physician for follow-up are imperative.

Onset. The onset of shock is characterized by few clinical signs. Signs or symptoms are rare until at least 10 per cent of the blood volume or 500 cc of systemic blood (for a man weighing 75 kg) is removed from the circulatory system. There may be a slight elevation of the diastolic blood pressure, indicative of the stress mechanism causing vasoconstriction. This stage is reversible.

Slight Degree of Shock. A slight degree of shock occurs with an average deficit of 1000 cc of blood or a blood pressure 20 per cent below normal. Many stress response symptoms are seen at this stage. Diastolic blood pressure may continue to be increased (vasoconstriction); pulse rate is increased (vasoconstriction and direct action of adrenalin on the myocardium); respiration rate is increased (resulting from presence of adrenalin); the skin is cool, pale, and dry (vasoconstriction); the basal metabolic rate is reduced (decreased volume). A patient in slight shock may be apprehensive (decreased blood volume to the brain) and may express listlessness and apathy. The patient in acute shock may experience fainting. As blood flow lessens, the patient may complain of weakness and dizziness; these may eventually result in unconsciousness. Painful stimuli may evoke only a groan or slightly defensive movements. The patient's urinary output will decrease. The laboratory test results on red blood cells may be normal, increased, or decreased, depending on the cause of shock. White blood cells may increase. Plasma proteins may decrease due to the passage of *protein-free interstitial fluid* into the blood from the interstitial spaces and intracellular fluids. The protein concentration in the blood has the ability to draw fluids from other compartments into the bloodstream when the hydrostatic pressure of the blood is down. Lactic acidosis occurs because of the incomplete oxidation of glucose. The blood urea nitrogen test reading is elevated due to decreased renal blood flow as well as increased breakdown of normal protein tissue. The blood sugar level is elevated as part of the stress response to the shock state. This stage is reversible.

Moderate Degree of Shock. A moderate degree of shock occurs with an average deficit of 1800 cc of blood or when the blood pressure is down 35 per cent from the normal. The symptoms of slight shock are aggravated. The pulse is still fast, but it may be weak, "thready," or irregular due to an insufficient supply of blood to the myocardium. Respiration is rapid and more shallow. The skin is pale, cool, and more clammy than in slight shock. The sensorium becomes duller with a progression to semiconsciousness. The pupils dilate and vision dims as less blood circulates to the brain. Oliguria becomes more pronounced.

Other stress compensations may come into play during this stage. The red bone marrow is stimulated by the hypoxia produced by the decreased blood volume. Mature red blood cells enter into the circulation to carry oxygen; when these are depleted, immature ones are released. This condition may be recognized by an increased reticulocyte count. Immature cells cannot carry as much oxygen as mature red blood cells, because they have less hemoglobin.

The liver and spleen release extra red blood cells.

The sympathoadrenal medullary responses (to stress) cause the kidneys to release a renal pressor substance **(RPS)** into the blood causing renal arteriolar vasoconstriction. This is also known as the vasoexcitor mechanism **(VEM).** RPS increases the tone of arterioles resulting in further arteriolar constriction.

Renin, a parahormone produced by an ischemic kidney, acts on plasma protein to form angiotonin which causes further vasoconstriction to increase the cardiac output.

Erthyropoietin, a parahormone that stimulates the production of red blood cells, is activated by the kidneys when they have been stimulated by the hypoxic state.

Release of the adrenocortical hormones is increased to further retain sodium and, therefore, water. This increases the blood volume, producing a higher cardiac output and better tissue perfusion.

This stage of shock is still reversible.

Severe Stage of Shock. The patient in the severe stage of shock enters a limbo where reversibility and irreversibility are not easily distinguishable. The severe stage of shock follows a 2500 cc loss of blood (for an average man weighing 75 kg) or a blood pressure decreased by 50 per cent. This is an acute condition. The vasoconstricting mechanisms are failing as evidenced by a dropping diastolic blood pressure and the collapse of veins. There is simply not enough blood available to expand the vessels. The pulse is rapid, but extremely thready and irregular; in most cases, it is barely perceptible. The nurse should take an apical pulse to determine the pulse rate. If the patient is on a monitor, arrhythmias may be noted due to decreased cardiac flow. Respiration is more shallow and rapid. The body may not be ridding itself of carbon dioxide fast enough, which further stimulates the respiratory center. The patient becomes unconscious due to acute hypoxia of the brain cells. The body's temperature-regulating mechanism may become disturbed. The skin is now ashen gray, cold, and clammy.

Frank cyanosis may be apparent. The degree of cyanosis is variable in each individual case. One determinative factor is the quantity of de-oxygenated hemoglobin in the artery which affects skin color, making it pale blue to dark bluish-red. A second determinative factor is the rate of blood flow through the skin. The pigmentation of the skin also affects the degree of cyanosis. The nurse should check light areas such as the lips and conjunctiva. Finally, the thickness of the skin alters the visibility of cyanosis. It is easier to see cyanosis in thin-skinned areas.

As the urine output decreases below 20 cc per hour to oliguria, the amount of tissue perfusion is greatly decreased. The prognosis becomes more negative if this situation is allowed to continue because kidney failure at this time is probably irreversible.

Table 18-1 summarizes the stages of shock and their characteristics.

Time is crucial in the recognition and treatment of the shock state. Shock is reversible if identified early and treated effectively. However, as cellular functions decrease, shock may become irreversible. To assure

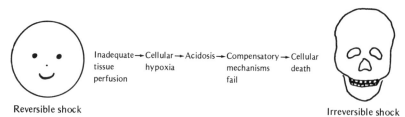

Reversible shock   Inadequate → Cellular → Acidosis → Compensatory → Cellular   Irreversible shock
                          tissue   hypoxia   mechanisms   death
                          perfusion   fail

Figure 18-6.   Continuum of shock.

TABLE 18-1. STAGES OF SHOCK AND THEIR CHARACTERISTICS

Stages of Shock	Blood Pressure	Fluid Vol. Deficit	Reversible/ Irreversible	Recognition	Potential Lab. Test Results*	Compensatory Mechanisms
Onset	Down 10%	500 cc	Rev.	Visible signs/symptoms rare; rise of diastolic blood pressure	None	Stress mechanism causing vasoconstriction
Slight	Down 20%	1,000 cc	Rev.	Diastolic blood pressure still increased; pulse rate increased; respirations increased; skin cool, pale, dry; basal metabolic rate reduced; listlessness, apathy, weakness, dizziness proceeding toward unconsciousness; decreasing urinary output	Red blood cells normal, decreased, or increased; white blood cells increased; plasma protein decreased; BUN increased; blood sugar increased	Stress mechanism releasing ACH; posterior pituitary releases ADH to hold water
Moderate	Down 35%	1,800 cc	Rev.	Fast pulse but weak and thready or irregular; respiration rapid and more shallow; skin pale, cool, clammy; sensorium dulled; dilating pupils; dim vision; oliguria	White blood cells increased; plasma protein decreased; BUN increased; blood sugar increased; hemoglobin and hematocrit may be increased, normal or decreased depending on cause of shock; red blood cells decreased in hemorrhage	Continuation of stress response; red bone marrow stimulated to release mature (and later immature) red blood cells into the system to carry oxygen; liver and spleen release extra red blood cells; kidneys release RPS to increase arteriolar constriction; renin acts on plasma protein to form angiotonin to further increase vasoconstriction;

TABLE 18-1. (continued)

				erythropoietin released by the kidneys to stimulate production of red blood cells; ACH released to retain sodium and thus water to increase blood volume
Severe	Down 50%	2,500 cc	Possibly irreversible	Diastolic blood pressure decreased; veins collapsing; pulse rapid, extremely thready and irregular, barely perceptible; arrhythmias appear on cardiac monitor; respiration rapid and more shallow; unconsciousness; peripheral skin ashen gray, cold, clammy; frank cyanosis; kidney failure (oliguria)	Serum sodium decreased; serum CO_2 decreased (acidosis); white blood cells increased; plasma protein decreased; BUN increased; blood sugar increased; hemoglobin and hematocrit may be increased, normal, or decreased depending on cause of shock; red blood cells decreased in hemorrhage	Stress mechanisms are failing; signs and symptoms point to cellular death

*All of these test results may not be seen in every individual. This is an inclusive guide.

optimal treatment, it is important that the nurse recognize signs and symptoms that indicate an improving as well as a deepening state of shock and then accurately and promptly report these signs to the physician. Shock is *preventable* and *reversible*. However, it is a continuum on which, as illustrated in Figure 18-6, *there is a point of no return.*

Factors That Increase the Severity of Shock

It is important for the nurse to be aware of situations that can aggravate an already critical state.

Extreme cold, below 28 degrees centigrade, will actually lead to gross peripheral vasodilation which decreases the amount of blood circulating in the bloodstream and thus to the vital organs. An example of this can be seen in the frostbite victim whose skin appears grossly reddened. A generalized mild coolness is compensatory until the body can replace the amount of blood lost or regain its vascular tone.

It is important that a person in shock become neither chilled nor too warm. Either extreme will hamper the effectiveness of vasoconstriction. What happens if hot water bottles and too many blankets are placed on the patient in shock? The heat causes peripheral vasodilation, drawing blood away from the systemic circulation. In addition, the hot water bottles are extremely dangerous, since a person in shock often loses peripheral neural sensations due to the decreased oxygenation of the skin. Thus, he may be burned without feeling it. If the patient is shivering, it is best to apply extra blankets, never hot water bottles. Shivering is an important sign because it indicates the patient is a step beyond just being cold. Also, shivering must be controlled, because it increases the body's metabolic rate. An increased rate of metabolism requires more oxygen, placing further demands on an already limited supply.

Severe pain may initiate or increase the severity of shock, because it may cause extreme vasoconstriction through increased stimulation of the sympathetic nervous system. Vasoconstriction, if not excessive, helps maintain and increase the circulating blood volume. However, severe vasoconstriction leads to further tissue hypoxia, reinforcing the necessary evil of shock. Thus, adequate relief of pain in the shock patient is important. However, the route of administration must be carefully selected. Intravenous infusion is the preferred method. If analgesics are administered intramuscularly or subcutaneously and the peripheral circulation is poor, very little of the drug may be absorbed. If, after several doses have been administered with little absorption, the shock state suddenly improves, with the resulting increased circulation, all the drugs may be absorbed at the same time. For example, if the patient has been given several doses of morphine, an improved shock state and restored circulation might result in an overdose of morphine, causing profound respiratory depression.

The duration of the shock will increase its severity: the longer the shock state, the greater the improper cellular metabolism, and thus the greater the accumulation of wastes to be excreted.

Anoxia, caused by other reasons than the shock, enhances a shock state. Anoxic anoxia (lack of oxygen), also called arterial anoxia, is due to respiratory obstruction, reduced oxygen supply in the air, or inadequate lung tissue across which sufficient oxygen may be diffused into the bloodstream. Because cellular oxygen in the victim of shock is already inadequate due to inadequate blood circulation or an inadequate blood volume, a diminished supply of oxygen to the blood further aggravates his shock state. This is why it is extremely important to maintain an un-obstructed airway and sufficient space for lung expansion in the patient in shock. Currently, the Trendelenburg position, previously thought to be the best position for a patient in shock, is being questioned because it forces the abdominal viscera up against the thoracic cavity, decreasing the space available for adequate lung expansion. An alternative position is the supine position in which only the feet are elevated. Adequate availability of oxygen is also important in a first aid situation, when it may be necessary to encourage a crowd to move away from the injured person to assure him access to the available oxygen.

Anemic anoxia is a deficiency of hemoglobin with a reduced number of red blood cells available to carry oxygen from the respiratory system, across the alveolus, to each cell of the body. Administration of oxygen to a patient in shock will be to no avail without sufficient hemoglobin to carry the extra oxygen to the cells.

Circulatory anoxia results from poor circulation of blood. Local anemia due to a decrease in arterial flow is called **ischemia.** Increased ischemia of tissues eventually leads to infarction, or death of tissue, from insufficient oxygen and nutrients. A decrease in venous flow is called stagnation. Stagnation leads to an accumulation of waste products (metabolic acidosis). Circulatory anoxia may be due to a weakened heart muscle or extremely viscous blood.

Histotoxic or metabolic anoxia occurs when the cells do not have the ability to utilize oxygen. An example of this is carbon monoxide poisoning.

Changes in the patient's position can also increase the severity of shock. Quick position changes will distort the tone of the peripheral blood vessels and may decrease the amount of blood returning to systemic circulation. For this reason, it is extremely important that a patient in shock be moved very evenly and slowly. It is best not to move him at all until his condition improves.

The presence of other diseases or disabling conditions in a patient may increase the difficulty of overcoming shock. For example, there is a decreased resistance to shock with age, hypoproteinemia, anemia, and malnutrition. It is interesting to note that females tolerate shock with or without blood loss better than males.

First Aid Care in Cases of Hemorrhage

In cases of hemorrhage, the initial objective of first aid care is to stop the flow of blood. This having been accomplished, the patient's blood loss can be replaced. Several first aid methods may be utilized.

It is important that rapid bleeding be stopped immediately. A pressure dressing or digital (finger-palm) pressure may be applied directly over the wound. In an emergency, a sterile dressing or clean hand is *not* the priority. Once a dressing has been applied it should not be removed, only reinforced, until the physician sees the patient. The dressing acts as a clot; if it is removed, the bleeding may resume.

Digital pressure against the artery proximal to the bleeding point will decrease the flow of blood so that clotting can take place. The blood flow is controlled by using the fingers or heel of the hand to press the supplying vessels against the underlying bone. The two main pressure points are the brachial and femoral arteries. Pressure on either will diminish the force of the blood flowing downward and thus assist clot formation. To occlude the brachial artery, apply pressure on the inner half of the arm midway between the elbow and the axilla. To occlude the femoral artery, apply pressure just below the groin on the front, inner half of the thigh, compressing the main vessel against the underlying pelvic bone.

Elevation of an extremity will also reduce the peripheral blood loss as well as shunt some peripheral blood to systemic circulation.

A tourniquet is used for severe bleeding that cannot be controlled by other means, as in the case of amputation.

Treatment and Nurse's Responsibilities

Because the responsibilities of the nurse and the treatment for shock are so closely aligned, they will be discussed together. Many of the nursing responsibilities regarding shock have been included in the foregoing discussions of a particular pathophysiology or treatment. Thus, parts of this list will be a review. Because this chapter has presented a great deal of information and guidelines regarding both the pathophysiology of shock and the keen observations required to deal with it, this brief summary of nursing responsibilities should aid you in organizing and assimilating this vital information.

Prevention of shock is most important and can be achieved through competent care. During surgery, the gentle handling of tissue, maintenance of complete homeostasis, immediate replacement of large losses of blood, minimal exposure of the viscera to atmospheric air, minimalization of the patient's apprehension and pain, careful anesthetization, effective postoperative care, and prompt treatment are the means available to prevent surgical shock. The nurse can be a valuable aid in alleviating the patient's anxiety preoperatively and in supporting the patient through the postoperative period.

Controlling hemorrhage is important.

Conservation of the patient's body heat with blankets is necessary, but not to the point of overheating the patient, thereby causing vasodilation. Remember to use shivering as a guide.

Do not unnecessarily move the patient as this may increase shock. By raising only the patient's feet, leaving the rest of his body in a supine position, approximately 500 cc of blood will be redirected to the circulatory system. The effect is one of giving an internal transfusion.

Judiciously relieve the pain. Pain intensifies shock.

Restlessness may indicate a need for oxygen.

Replace required fluids.

The primary objective of the health team is the prevention of irreversible shock. The overall objective of treatment and nursing care as well as of all the body's compensatory mechanisms is to restore or maintain adequate tissue perfusion for the maximal resistance of the patient to shock.

CASE STUDY 18 *

A 58-year-old man was admitted to the hospital with a diagnosis of intestinal obstruction. Following surgery, he developed persistent vomiting. A Levin tube was inserted and connected to Gomco suction. Gastric drainage was between 100 and 3500 cc/24 hours for the next week.

*For answers to Case Study Questions, see Appendix 4.

Questions

1. What electrolyte imbalance(s) could develop from gastric drainage?

2. A patient on gastric suction loses approximately _____ mEq/L sodium, _____ mEq/L chloride, and _____ mEq/L potassium.

3. Ten days following surgery, the nurses were six liters behind on the administration of intravenous fluids, and the patient began hemorrhaging in the surgical area. He became restless, cold, sweaty, his pulse increased, and his blood pressure dropped. Blood transfusions were ordered to run continuously, but the patient did not respond. What is the nurse's responsibility at this point?

4. The patient was returned to surgery to control bleeding, but his condition still did not improve as desired. He developed diaphoresis, and his vital signs remained unstable. What is the significance of diaphoresis?

5. The patient's condition continued to deteriorate, and he developed hypovolemic shock and oliguria. Why did the physician order Mannitol to be given by intravenous injection?

The patient did not respond to the Mannitol, and it was determined that he had developed acute renal failure (acute tubular necrosis) from poor perfusion of the kidneys.

6. Evaluate the following laboratory test results:
Na 122 mEq/L; Cl 86 mEq/L; CO_2 9 mEq/L; pH 7.20; BUN 188 mg %; and creatinine 10 mg %.

Case Summary: The patient's family decided against hemodialysis for treatment of the acute renal failure.

In summary, this patient progressively developed: hypovolemia, shock, oliguria, acute renal failure, uremia, death.

Quiz 18*

A 58-year-old man was admitted to the hospital with a diagnosis of intestinal obstruction. Following surgery, a Levin tube was inserted and connected to Gomco suction because of persistent vomiting. He subsequently had large amounts of gastric drainage. He hemorrhaged, developed a shock condition, became oliguric, and suffered acute renal failure and renal metabolic acidosis.

Check the following as either true or false:

True	False	
_____	_____	1. Marked increase or decrease of nasogastric suction (increased or decreased by 500 cc/shift) should be reported to the physician.
_____	_____	2. Levin tubes should be irrigated with 30 cc sterile water.
_____	_____	3. The majority of shock patients need volume replacement.
_____	_____	4. Blood pressure is a reliable guide to tissue perfusion.
_____	_____	5. Urinary output is a reliable guide to tissue perfusion.
_____	_____	6. As long as the blood pressure did not continue to drop, the nurse could assume the patient was "holding his own."
_____	_____	7. Decreased urinary output could be the first indication of impending renal failure.
_____	_____	8. Mannitol is an osmotic diuretic.
_____	_____	9. Poor perfusion of kidneys from shock caused this patient to develop renal failure.
_____	_____	10. All patients with renal failure should be placed on an artificial kidney.

BIBLIOGRAPHY

American Red Cross: First Aid Text, 1972.
Beland, I., and Passos, J. Y.: Clinical Nursing: Pathophysiological and Psychological Approaches, ed. 3. The Macmillan Company, New York, 1975.
Bordicks, K. J.: Patterns of Shock. Implications for Nursing Care, ed. 2. The Macmillan Company, New York, 1970.

*For answers to Quizzes, see Appendix 5.

Bradley, E. C. and Weil, M. H.: Treatment of circulatory shock with adrenolytic (vasodilator) drug. Clin. Res. 13:120, 1965.

Brooks, D. K., Williams, W. G., Manley, R. W., and Whiteman, P.: Osmolar and electrolyte changes in haemorrhagic shock. Hypertonic solutions in the prevention of tissue damage. Lancet 1:521, 1963.

Brunner, L., et al.: Textbook of Medical-Surgical Nursing, ed. 2. J. B. Lippincott Company, Philadelphia, 1970.

Burrell, L. O., and Burrell, Z. L., Jr.: Intensive Nursing Care. The C. V. Mosby Company, St. Louis, 1969.

Condon, R. E., and Nyhus, L. M.: Manual of Surgical Therapeutics, ed. 3. Little, Brown and Company, Boston, 1975.

Grove, L.: The microcirculation and shock. J. Am. Assoc. Nurse Anesth. 40:105, 1972.

Guntheroth, W. G., Abel, F. L., and Mullins, G. L.: The effect of Trendelenburg's position on blood pressure and carotid flow. Surg. Gynecol. Obstet. 119:345, 1964.

Guyton, A. C.: Textbook of Medical Physiology, ed. 5. W. B. Saunders Company, Philadelphia, 1976.

Hershey, S. G., Mazzia, V. D. B., Altura, B. M., and Gyure, L.: Effects of vasopressors on the microcirculation and on survival in hemorrhagic shock. Anesthesiology 26:179, 1965.

Hume, D. M., and Nelson, D. H.: Adrenal cortical function in surgical shock. Surg. Forum 5:568, 1964.

Lillehei, R. C., et al.: Treatment of septic shock. Mod. Treat. 4:321, 1967.

Mason, E. E.: Fluid, Electrolyte, and Nutrient Therapy in Surgery. Lea and Febiger, Philadelphia, 1974.

Metheny, N. M., and Snively, W. D., Jr.: Nurses' Handbook of Fluid Balance, ed. 2. J. B. Lippincott Company, Philadelphia, 1974.

Mills, L. J., and Moyer, J. H. (eds.): Shock and Hypotension — Pathogenesis and Treatment. Grune and Stratton, Inc., New York, 1965.

Modern Concept of Shock. The Upjohn Company, Kalamazoo, Michigan, 1967.

Porter, R., and Knight, J.: Energy Metabolism in Trauma. CIBA Foundation, Churchhill, London, 1970.

Smith, S. E.: Drug therapy 1972. 4. Diuretic drugs. Nurs. Times 68:349, 1972.

Thal, A. P., and Wilson, R.: Shock, Current Problems in Surgery. Year Book Medical Publishers, Inc., Chicago, 1965.

Weil, M. H. and Shubin, H.: Diagnosis and Treatment of Shock. The Williams and Wilkins Company, Baltimore, 1967.

NOTES

NOTES

19

Burns

Burns are particularly critical in regard to fluid and electrolyte balance because they present an immediate danger to life. The greatest threats to a burn patient are shock and renal failure as a result of extensive fluid loss. Since approximately 10,000 hospital beds are occupied by burn patients each year and approximately 7,000 people die annually from burn-related injuries the need to know burn therapy is vital.

Types

Burns may be due to thermal, chemical or electrical injury. The most common incidents of burns are caused by sunburn; scalds; direct contact with flame; strong acids, alkalis or corrosive fluids; powder burns; electricity; and inhalation of heat and smoke. Decubiti and excessive skin reaction to radiation therapy can also be considered as a form of burn.

Burn Evaluation

There is no system for evaluation of the extent of burns that measures precisely the amount of fluid lost by a burn victim. However, since it is so important to replace fluids immediately a simple though somewhat imprecise method has been devised. Two factors must be considered when estimating the burn patient's fluid replacement. One is the amount of surface involvement and the other is the depth of the burn. The Rule of Nines and the Lund and Browder chart provide approximate guides to determining surface involvement in percent of total body surface area.

The Rule of Nines divides the body on a rough visual basis into multiples of 9 per cent (Fig. 19–1).

The Lund and Browder chart gives a more extensive breakdown of areas of the body and also distinguishes between different age groups (Fig. 19 – 2).

As stated previously, the depth as well as the surface area of a burn is important in determining fluid loss. Burn depth is classified by degree. *First degree burns* are indicated by dry, red skin. There are no blisters. This type of burn is minor unless the age factor causes it to be more critical. Although a first degree burn is painful it usually heals itself unless the patient is a young child or an adult over 65 years of age. The most common cause of first degree burn is overexposure to the sun, sunburn.

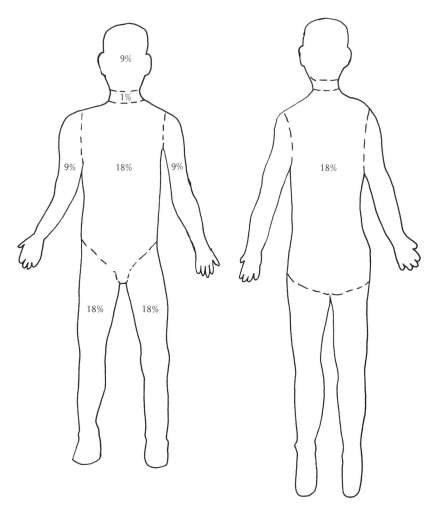

Figure 19-1. Rule of Nines: Head 9%; Neck 1%; Each entire arm 9% (front only 4½%); Front 18%; Back 18%; Each entire leg 18% (front only 9%).

In second degree burns the skin is red, wet and blistered. A *second degree burn* is very painful but will usually heal itself if not complicated by infection. Scalding with hot liquids is considered the primary cause of second degree burns.

Third degree burns are the most serious. The skin is dry, frequently with a leathery eschar or slough. Charred blood vessels may be visible beneath the eschar. The skin color may be white or dark colored and charred. There is little or no pain. Skin grafting is required for the burned area to heal. Third degree burns are usually caused by direct contact with flame, chemicals or electricity.

Not only are they classified as first, second or third degree but burns also may be described as minor or major. A *minor burn* is one that covers a small area of the body, less than 9 per cent in an adult. The skin is reddened, unbroken and exhibits no blisters. A *major burn* is one which covers 9 per cent of the total body surface area (TBSA). In a major burn the skin is both broken and blistered.

LUND AND BROWDER CHART								
	Age -- Years					%	%	%
Area	0-1	1-4	5-9	10-15	Adult	2°	3°	Total
Head	19	17	13	10	7			
Neck	2	2	2	2	2			
Ant. trunk	13	17	13	13	13			
Post. trunk	13	13	13	13	13			
R. buttock	2½	2½	2½	2½	2½			
L. buttock	2½	2½	2½	2½	2½			
Genitalia	1	1	1	1	1			
R. U. Arm	4	4	4	4	4			
L. U. Arm	4	4	4	4	4			
R. L. Arm	3	3	3	3	3			
L. L. Arm	3	3	3	3	3			
R. Hand	2½	2½	2½	2½	2½			
L. Hand	2½	2½	2½	2½	2½			
R. Thigh	5½	6½	8½	8½	9½			
L. Thigh	5½	6½	8½	8½	9½			
R. Leg	5	5	5½	6	7			
L. Leg	5	5	5½	6	7			
R. Foot	3½	3½	3½	3½	3½			
L. Foot	3½	3½	3½	3½	3½			
					Total			

Figure 19-2.   Reprinted from Initial Burn Management, Flint Laboratories, Division of Travenol Laboratories, Inc., Deerfield, Ill., 1975, with permission.

Pathophysiology

The pathophysiology of severe burn trauma involves rapid fluid and electrolyte changes. There is an apparent redistribution of fluid, protein and minerals as they accumulate in and around the thermally injured tissues but it has not been determined how this anatomically occurs. Fluid accumulates in interstitial spaces and/or in blisters. The latter type of accumulation is a third space fluid loss. Fluid is also lost as a result of evaporation. Loss due to evaporation is called "white bleeding." Both types of fluid loss deplete the circulating fluid volume and can precipitate hypovolemic shock.

A redistribution or loss of other components of the body chemistry occurs along with the fluid loss. Large amounts of sodium move with the fluid from the intravascular to the interstitial fluid area during the first 24 hours. At this time the patient usually is oliguric. Potassium becomes elevated in the bloodstream owing to the destruction of tissue and oliguria. The result of this shift is hyperkalemia.

It is believed that the entire sequestration of isotonic fluid and body chemicals occurs within the first 24 hours, a situation which causes saline deficit and possibly leads to hypovolemic shock.

During the second 24 hours postburn the sodium shifts back from the interstitial space into the intravascular. The patient then begins to diurese and may move into hypokalemia as a consequence of potassium lost via the urine. Other electrolytes, most significantly magnesium and serum proteins, are also lost and vitamin deficiencies caused by lack of intake are also common. There is red blood cell loss from a microangiopathic anemia. The seriousness of this anemia is correlated to the severity and extent of the burn. Red blood cell destruction is caused initially by the heat of the burn and later by hemolysis of heat-damaged cells. A shift in the pH balance is another change which occurs in the body chemistry. Acidosis appears as the kidney function decreases and uremic waste products are retained. Rapid destruction of body cells causes the release of intracellular potassium which results in hyperkalemia. Further intensification of hyper-kalemia is caused by oliguria.

After 48 hours the blood volume becomes expanded because of the edema fluid mobilization; this results in saline excess and circulatory over-load. Fluid mobilization may cause clinical signs and laboratory values to be deceptive. Examples of such deceptive indications of improvement are high cardiac output and diuresis.

Part of the devastation caused by burns is due to related factors which increase the severity of burns. The possibility of hypovolemic shock in-creases as the destruction of tissue increases. The mortality rate is high when massive tissue destruction covers 65 per cent of the TBSA. Age is also a factor; mortality rate is increased in the aged and infants. Infection is particularly difficult to control in the burn patient.

Curling's or peptic ulcers may develop because of the severe stress. Therefore, gastric mucosal irritation or injury should be recognized and should be prevented with nasogastric suction, antacids and adequate nutri-tional support. Surgery is usually indicated if gastrointestinal hemorrhage cannot be controlled by medical procedures.

Respiratory distress is another complication in burn patients. It is often difficult to distinguish the respiratory effects of hypovolemic shock from lung injury. Lung injuries can be differentiated from hypovolemic shock by the presence of rhonci and rales. Death is often the result of pulmonary interstitial edema related to the hypovolemic shock.

Bacterial pneumonia is another factor which limits survival. Another complication of burn shock is acute renal failure.

The return of optimal function of the burned areas requires many months and frequently many years. This is especially true of the extremities, neck and axillae. Immediate skilled attention by the health team and procedures such as surgery skin grafting, and the relief of contractures maximize the burn patient's chance of survival and his return to optimal functions.

Treatment

Burn treatment will be discussed in terms of first aid, emergency room treatment and finally the more extensive treatment of fluid replacement and compensation for loss of life-sustaining functions.

First Aid

The most urgent concern of anyone on the scene of a fire is to remove the burn victim from contact with whatever is causing the burn. If the victim is on fire force him to lie flat and roll him in a blanket or coat. This will smother the flames. Immediately apply cool water to the burn area. Cool water will help ease the pain, prevent afterglow, constrict the blood vessels and help remove the irritating substance from the skin if the burn is due to chemicals.

No greasy ointments, butter, lard or other dressings should be applied. Such applications retain the heat in the burn and thus increase tissue damage. Greasy applications also interfere with other necessary forms of treatment and enhance the possibility of infection. However, do cover the burn with a clean sheet. The sheet may be wet with cool tap water. The sheet will help prevent contamination, thus decreasing the chances of infection, and will alleviate some of the victims discomfort due to air currents.

Establish an adequate airway. When emergency personnel are available more indepth evaluation of the burn victim should occur. A tracheotomy is not necessary for every patient with a head or neck burn but preparation should be made. Later indications that a tracheotomy may be necessary are increased hoarseness, changes in respiratory pattern and/or a sudden increase in laryngeal secretions. An endotracheal tube should be used first for about five days if intubation is necessary.

Apply pressure to stop the bleeding.

Start Ringer's Lactate I.V. if it will require more than thirty minutes to transport the patient to the hospital.

Transport to the hospital as quickly as possible.

Emergency Room Care

Irrigate the burned area with normal saline as soon as the patient is admitted to the emergency room. If possible give the patient a shower. This is especially applicable for patients with chemical burns. Alkali burns need not be treated with diluted acid.

Further cleanse the burned area with cool water and bland soap. Remove all dirt and loose skin. Shave the surrounding normal skin and scalp. Blisters form an ideal protective shield against infection and against fluid loss from white bleeding and they should not be broken.

Immobilize the burned parts. If the hands are burned wrap them in a position of function.

Perform the initial venipuncture and establish a reliable intravenous site. Once the needs of the patient have been assessed, plan and implement the following procedures: pain medication, tetanus prophylaxis, antibiotics, and fluid replacement.

Determine the need for nasogastric tube and Foley catheter. Insert if needed.

Emotional reassurance is important since anxiety can increase the possibility of shock.

A check list for emergency management is given in Table 19 – 1.

Burn Unit Care

After the initial emergency procedures have been completed it is vital that an evaluation be made of the extracellular fluid volume changes. The amount of fluid replacement should be calculated from the time of the burn. The calculated loss should be replaced within the first 24 hours in burns covering 20 per cent or more of the TBSA. This aggressive administration of biologically active fluid in the first 24 hours will usually maintain circulatory integrity and prevent visceral failure and subsequent death.

It is considered advisable to have several alternative methods of fluid replacement to suit the physiological function of the individual. The use of

TABLE 19-1.   EMERGENCY MANAGEMENT

do's	dont's
Obtain history.	NO salves or ointments.
Give morphine I. V.	DON'T perform tracheostomy unless
Check for obstructed airway.	absolutely necessary.
Perform initial venipuncture.	NO pain medication I. M.
Insert indwelling urinary catheter.	In severe burns, DON'T give water orally
Establish a reliable I. V. portal.	(may induce vomiting)
Determine need for nasogastric tube.	
Check for other injuries.	
Estimate extent of injury. (Rule of Nines)	
Give tetanus prophylaxis.	
Determine need for antibiotics.	
Plan fluid replacement therapy.	
Consider special nurses, critical list, and	
blood donors.	
Make worksheet.	

NOTE: Chemical and electrical burns generally require more attention.

Reprinted from Initial Burn Management, Flint Laboratories, Division of Travenol Laboratories, Inc., Deerfield, Ill., 1975, with permission.

TABLE 19-2.   THREE MAJOR REGIMENS FOR FLUID REPLACEMENT

The Brooke Formula	The Evans Formula
During first 24 hours:	During first 24 hours:
Colloids (blood, dextran or plasma):	*Colloids:*
0.5 ml. per kg. per per cent of body surface burned.	1 ml. per kg. per per cent of body surface burned.
Lactated Ringer's solution:	*Physiologic saline solution:*
1.5 ml. per kg. per per cent of body surface burned.	1 ml. per kg. per per cent of body surface burned.
Water requirement (dextrose in water):	*Nonelectrolytes:*
2000 ml. for adults; correspondingly less in children.	2000 ml. of 5 per cent dextrose in water; correspondingly less in children.
If, in a burn of more than 50 per cent in a large patient, fluid therapy based on a 50 per cent restriction fails to prevent signs and symptoms of circulatory failure, therapy must be cautiously increased. One half of the estimated fluid requirements for the first 24 hours is usually given in the first 8 hours, one fourth in the second 8 hours, and one fourth in the third 8 hours.	

The Parkland Regimen:

During first 24 hours:

Lactated Ringer's solution is given in the amount of 4 ml. per kg. per per cent of body surface burned.

NOTE: In adults, maintain urine output at 30 to 50 cc. per hour.

more crystalloid and less colloid replacement is appearing in the burn regimen each year.

Currently there are three major regimens for fluid replacement: The Brooke Formula, the Evans Formula and the Parkland Regimen (Table 19 – 2).

Following immediate postburn massive intravenous fluid and electrolyte therapy, it is imperative that the patient's increased nutritional needs be met. A high protein, high calorie diet accompanied by vitamins should be given as soon as possible. Burned adults require about 60 calories per kilogram of body weight and about 3 gram of protein per kilogram of body weight. Children usually require approximately 85 calories per kilogram of body weight and 4 gram of protein per kilogram of body weight. Administer, as appropriate, large amounts of ascorbic acid, the B vitamins and the fat soluble vitamins A, D, and K.

Since infection frequently accompanies burns, antibiotics may be prescribed. Penicillin and streptomycin are frequently used for the first three to five days and then discontinued. They may be resumed later following debridement or to treat cellulitis and septicemia.

Topical agents which may be applied are silver nitrate, Sulfamylon, Silvadene and Betadine. However, avoid early application of such agents as they compound the metabolic acidosis of the shock phase.

Pain is another important factor to be considered in planning the treatment procedure for a burn patient. Some relief from pain is usually administered during the initial emergency treatment. Never give pain medication intramuscularly. Owing to poor circulation it may not be absorbed into the bloodstream. A build up of pain medication due to IM administration could cause an overdose when normal circulation is restored.

Morphine may be administered intravenously, especially if the burn covers more than 20 per cent of the TBSA. Large doses of narcotics should be avoided, especially in children. Patient restlessness in the acute phase is frequently due to hypovolemia or hypoxia and not pain.

Follow-up Care

Having stabilized the patient's body fluids and electrolytes and performed other procedures, the health team needs to determine whether the patient can be treated as an outpatient or whether further hospitalization is necessary.

If outpatient status is selected, cover the burn site with a thick, fluffy dressing followed by a fine mesh gauze. The patient should be instructed how and when to change the dressing at home. Antibiotics are not usually prescribed unless cellulitis develops.

Patients who are capable of self-care with first degree burns covering less than 15 per cent of the TBSA can usually be placed on outpatient status.

Hospitalization is usually indicated in the following situations: if the patient has second degree burns involving more than 15 per cent of the TBSA; if there are third degree burns with a TBSA involvement of more than 3 per cent; if there are lesser burns in children and the aged; if patients with a history of asthma or diabetes have 5 per cent burn areas; or if there are lesser degree burns that involve the hands, feet, face and perineum.

Other considerations besides the degree of burn involvement are lung injury, high voltage electrical injury, chemical burns of the eyes, patients with sickle cell anemia, suspected battered children and parents incapable of handling the situation because of a number of other small children.

Tissue treatment may be a factor in requiring hospitalization. Escharotomy and fasciotomy may need to be performed. These are usually performed to full-thickness (all layers of skin inclusive) circumferential burns between one to three days after the burn. An escharotomy will help maintain adequate circulation to an area. This procedure may be performed at the bedside. It is a lateral process requiring no anesthesia. A fasciotomy is frequently performed on high voltage electrical injuries. Generally it is indicated if the vascular compression is not relieved by the escharotomy. An example of a typical fasciotomy is that performed in the case of a compressed anterior tibial, indicated by loss of foot sensation and footdrop.

Because of infection and the lack of proper blood circulation to the tissue, necrotic tissue may develop. Chemical debridement can be initiated two to five days postburn. Travase is an example of an effective enzyme for burn debridement. Travase has also been used successfully in the debridement of decubiti ulcers. It dissolves necrotic tissue and purulent exudates.

Excision of full-thickness burns permits the patient to regain early motion and rapid return of functions. Nonviable tendons are excised at this time. There are two procedures used to excise burns. One is performed with a cold knife; the bleeding is usually profuse. A single thickness (ST) skin graft is stored and applied two days later. Electrosurgical excision is the second method to excise burns. It is performed from three to thirteen days postburn. The procedure is followed by topical silver nitrate therapy. Electrosurgical excision with immediate skin graft is reported to achieve good results.

Early removal of necrotic tissue and closure of burn wounds appears to contribute to the survival of the patient.

Nurse's Responsibilities

Because burn patients are in a state of rapid fluctuation, nursing care is important throughout every stage of the burn patient's recovery.

Monitor vital signs.

Maintain accurate intake and output records because urine output is the best guide to the patient's fluid status and the possibility of hypovolemic shock.

Prevent shock by administering calculated fluid loss I.V. This is particularly important during the first 24 hours postburn.

Conserve the patient's body heat to prevent lactic acidosis caused by the increased oxygen consumption and the resulting inadequate metabolism of carbohydrates.

Administer pain medication I.V. as needed.

Be alert to changes in respiratory pattern since changes may be indicative of inhalation injury or pulmonary edema.

Maintain sterility of wounds and asepsis of environment.

Meet the increased nutritional needs of the patient by increasing the amounts of protein, calories and vitamins.

Maintain a patent I.V. mainline.

Be alert to psychological and emotional needs.

BIBLIOGRAPHY

Anderson, L., et al.: Nutrition in Nursing. J. B. Lippincott Company, Philadelphia, 1972.

Baxter, C. R.: Management of fluid volume and electrolyte changes in the early postburn period. Geriatrics 30: 57, 1975.

Bergersen, B. S.: Pharmacology in Nursing. The C. V. Mosby Company, St. Louis, 1973.

Czaja, A. J., et al.: Acute gastric disease after cutaneous thermal injury. Arch. Surg. 110: 600, 1975.

Dudrick, S. J., et al.: Long-term total parenteral nutrition with growth, development, and positive nitrogen balance. Surgery 64: 134, 1968.

Goodman, L., and Gilman, A.: The Pharmacological Basis of Therapeutics. The Macmillan Company, New York, 1970.

Initial Burn Management. Flint Laboratories, Division of Travenol Laboratories, Inc., Deerfield, Illinois, 1975.

Lewis, R. J., and Quinby, W. C.: Electrosurgical excision of full-thickness burns. Arch. Surg. 110: 191, 1975.

Polk, H. C., and Stone, H. H.: Contemporary Burn Management. Little, Brown and Company, Boston, 1971.

Stephenson, S. F., Esrig, B. C., and Polk, H. C.: The pathophysiology of smoke inhalation injury. Ann. Surg. 182: 652, 1975.

192

NOTES

SECTION VI

NURSING TECHNIQUES

20

Peritoneal Dialysis

Peritoneal dialysis is a procedure with two main objectives: to remove toxic substances from the body and to remove excess fluids, restoring the proper electrolyte balance. The presence of toxic substances may be due to ingestion or may result from an inability of the kidneys to excrete the metabolic waste products.

The following are the more common conditions in which peritoneal dialysis could be indicated:

intoxication from dialyzable poisons or drugs;

acute renal failure due to shock;

hemolysis caused by a mismatched blood transfusion;

chronic renal failure involving a sudden loss of therapeutic control in primary renal disease;

transplant preparation;

electrolyte, acid-base, or fluid imbalance.

Conditions where peritoneal dialysis could be contraindicated include the following:

abdominal adhesions causing functional impediments;

severe abdominal trauma;

aortic surgeries and grafts;

presence of coagulation defects.

Peritoneal dialysis can be used alone or as a supportive measure between extracorporeal hemodialysis procedures.

Principles of Dialysis

Peritoneal dialysis is accomplished by osmosis and diffusion. A dialysate solution is instilled into the abdominal cavity where it is retained for 60 to 90 minutes until the toxic substances have time to diffuse across the peritoneal membrane into the dialysate. The fluid is then drained off, taking excess fluid and toxic waste products with it. Excess fluids are removed by osmosis, whereas the larger molecular waste products, such as urea and creatinine, are removed by diffusion. Molecules which are too large to pass through the membrane are, of course, retained by the body.

The composition of the peritoneal dialysis solution is essentially the same as normal serum in mEq/L with three exceptions: First, bicarbonate is replaced with 45 mEq/L of lactate in the dialysate solution because it is more stable. Second, potassium is omitted or added separately as the physician determines the patient's need. Third is the addition of a larger amount of glucose. Normal serum contains 1 gm/L of glucose, whereas the most frequently used dialysate solution contains 15 gm/L or 1.5 per cent glucose. When it is necessary to remove excess fluid, a dialysate solution of 70 gm/L or 7 per cent glucose should be used. As with all medications, the solution label should be conscientiously checked to avoid confusing the 7 per cent with the 1.5 per cent solution. When using a high dextrose concentration, close monitoring of the patient's volume status and blood sugar level is required. Excessive fluid removal can cause hypovolemia and endanger the patient's life; for this reason, 7 per cent solutions of glucose should be administered cautiously. Seven per cent solution is usually used in conjunction with one liter of 7 per cent glucose and one liter of 1.5 per cent glucose. Even then, it is not usually used for more than one exchange.

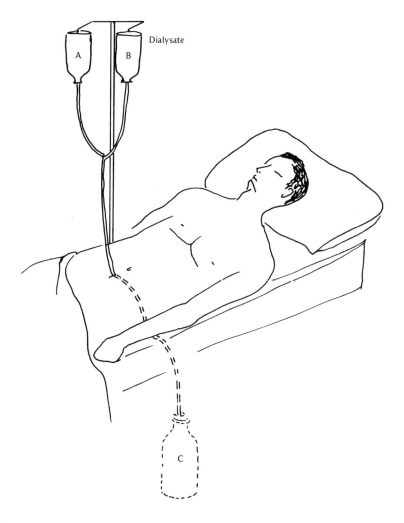

Figure 20-1.   Peritoneal dialysis. Dialysate (A and B) is infused into the peritoneum; waste products diffuse across the peritoneal membrane to the dialysate; dialysate return is evacuated into bottle (C).

Procedure

Peritoneal dialysis is initiated as a minor surgical procedure usually performed in the patient's bed. The procedure is relatively simple, inexpensive, and available. Complete dialysis kits are now easily obtained from surgical supply companies.

Because the nurse plays a major role in the dialysis procedure, it is essential that she have a working knowledge of electrolyte and fluid balance.

Preparation. The nurse may be requested to explain the dialysis procedure to the patient and his family, and to obtain a permit if one is required by the hospital. In preparation for peritoneal dialysis, the nurse should request the patient to empty his bladder if an indwelling catheter is not present, obtain his vital signs, and record an accurate balance-scale weight.

A sedative should be administered if ordered by the physician. Heparin should be available for addition to dialysate solution as deemed necessary by the physician to prevent blood clotting in the peritoneal catheter.

Technique.

1. Warm the prepared dialysate solution to 38° C (100.4°F).
2. Cleanse the abdominal area, and prepare a sterile field.
3. Open the sterile dialysis kit.
4. The physician will insert a catheter, by rotating it in through a stab wound at a point one-third the distance from umbilicus to pubis.
5. Position the catheter, and secure it with sutures or tape.
6. Attach the connection hook-up, as shown in Figure 20-1.
7. Maintain a flow sheet, recording the intake and output of all exchanges.

PERITONEAL DIALYSIS RECORD SHEET

Name: Doe, Jane   Date: 1-2-74

Hospital No.: 123-456-789   Diagnosis: Acute renal failure (ECF excess, hyperkalemia)

Age: 36   Weight (baseline): 115 lbs.

Time	No.	Volume In	Volume Out	Fluid Balance	Medication	Remarks
9:00 A	1	2000			1.5% Dialysate Solution	Vital Signs BP 130/70 P100 R24
9:40	1		1800	+200		Drainage slightly sanguineous
10:00	2	2000			Same	
10:40	2		1700	+500		Less sanguineous
11:00	3	2000			4.25% Dialysate Solution	
11:40	3		2400	+100		
12:00P	4	2000			1.5% Dialysate Solution	VS BP 128/64 P98 R20
12:40	4		2000	+100		
1:00	5	2000			Same	
1:40	5		2200	-100		Drainage slowed - catheter
2:00	6	2000			Same	adjusted
2:40	6		1900	0		Abdominal pain during
3:00	7	2000			Same	drainage - 5cc 2%
3:40	7		2100	+100		Procaine into catheter

Figure 20-2. Sample peritoneal dialysis record sheet.

Each exchange takes approximately an hour. The 2000 cc of dialysate solution will usually run into the peritoneum in 20 minutes. The tubes are then clamped, and the solution is allowed to remain in the abdominal cavity for 20 minutes. The lower clamps are then opened to allow the fluid to drain into the lower bottle. This process takes approximately 20 minutes. The procedure is repeated each hour for as many exchanges as the physician orders, usually over a period of 24 to 48 hours.

Nurse's Responsibilities

The nurse is responsible for maintaining an accurate record on the flow sheet of the precise time, composition, and amount of dialysate solution intake and output on all exchanges. See Fig. 20-2 for a sample flow record sheet. The patient undergoing peritoneal dialysis requires continuous and skillful care. Every effort should be made to keep him as comfortable as possible. Meals should be scheduled when the abdomen is empty of dialysate fluid. The patient is usually more comfortable if the backrest is elevated. Changing the patient's position will often facilitate drainage of the dialysate solution. Vital signs should be taken as often as the patient's condition indicates. Since each bottle of dialysate fluid does not contain exactly one liter, the nurse should occasionally check the patient's body weight with a bed scale when the dialysate has been drained off.

BIBLIOGRAPHY

Davidson, R. C., and Scribner, B. H.: A Physician's Syllabus for the Treatment of Chronic Uremia. University of Washington, Seattle, 1967.

Maxwell, M. H., et al. Peritoneal dialysis; 1. Technique and applications. J.A.M.A. 170:917, 1959.

Papper, S.: Clinical Nephrology. Little, Brown and Company, Boston, 1971.

Twiss, M. R., and Maxwell, M. H.: Peritoneal dialysis. Am. J. Nurs. 59:1560, 1959.

NOTES

NOTES

21

Hemodialysis

Extracorporeal hemodialysis is a technique of filtering the patient's blood outside the body using an artificial kidney. The purposes of hemodialysis are the same as for peritoneal dialysis: to remove toxic products, both chemical and metabolic, and to remove excess fluid and correct electrolyte imbalances. Hemodialysis is usually used when the patient's condition cannot be maintained by more conservative therapy. The patient's clinical condition chiefly determines whether or not to perform hemodialysis. Extracorporeal hemodialysis is a faster and more efficient method than peritoneal dialysis for removing urea and other toxic products.

There are several different types of artificial kidney machines. The Kolff and the Kiil are two of the more common types currently available. Although some of the machines are becoming quite sophisticated with automatic devices and alarm systems, the basic principles and components of the machines are essentially the same. Most of the systems include the use of dialysate solution and consist of a large vat, a cellophane coil, connecting tubes, a circulating pump and a blood pump (see Figure 21-1).

The dialysate concentrate is poured into the vat and diluted according to the physician's directions, and the coil and tubings are primed, freed of air, and checked for leakage. The arterial line of the patient's shunt is connected by tubing to the coil. The placement of the arteriovenous shunt requires a rather long and tedious surgical procedure. This is one of the reasons more conservative methods of treatment are preferred over hemodialysis.

The type of shunt used varies according to whether the patient has an acute or chronic condition. In acute conditions, a shunt with silastic tubing is placed into an artery and a vein. A plastic connector hooks them together outside the body. They are separated for connection to the artificial kidney and reconnected for the resumption of normal blood flow.

In chronic conditions requiring long-term hemodialysis, the arteriovenous (AV) fistula is the preferred method of shunting. An artery and vein are grafted together and remain under the skin. After a ''ripening'' period in which the graft is allowed to enlarge through the process of a back flow of venous blood into the artery, the shunt is ready for use. The patient is connected to the machine for each procedure by two needle placements similar to those used in venipuncture.

Once the shunt is connected, the pump draws the blood into the coil. The

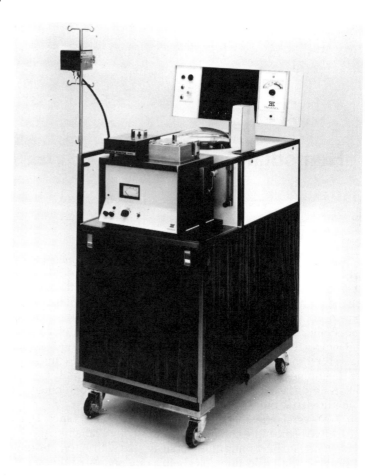

Figure 21-1. RSP artificial kidney. (Courtesy of Travenol Laboratories, Inc., Artificial Organs Division, Morton Grove, Illinois 60053).

coil is composed of cellophane wound inside a plastic mesh (see Figure 21-2). The cellophane is the semipermeable membrane necessary for the osmosis and diffusion of the toxic materials into the dialysate. The dialysate solution is circulated around the cellophane in the coil by the action of the circulating pump. During this action, the excess fluid and waste products are extracted from the blood. When the blood leaves the coil, it is returned to the patient through the venous line of the shunt. This procedure usually requires four to eight hours and is repeated two or three times a week.

Conditions requiring extracorporeal hemodialysis fall into two general categories: acute and chronic. Acute conditions include overdoses of drugs or poisons, trauma due to crushing injuries or shock, hemolysis, and pancreatitis. Patients with an acute condition who are using an artificial kidney require extremely skilled nursing care. Patients with acute conditions have a high mortality rate. In many cases, acute renal failure is reversed, but 30 to 50 per cent of these patients die from other causes, such as injuries or septicemia.

Many patients with chronic renal diseases are maintained by a controlled diet alone and function very well. There are many, however, whose kidney function is so greatly diminished that they must be maintained on an artificial kidney in order to sustain life.

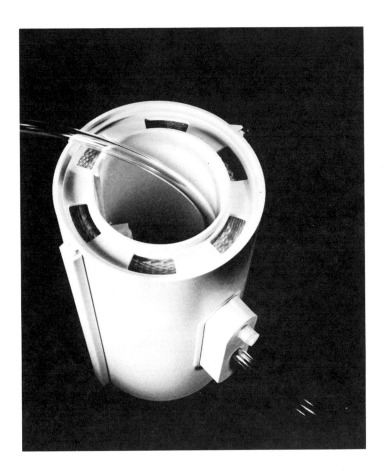

Figure 21-2.   Ultra-Flo 11 coil dialyzer. (Courtesy of Travenol Laboratories, Inc., Artificial Organs Division, Morton Grove, Illinois 60053.)

A criterion must be established for the selection of patients requiring extracorporeal hemodialysis. Selection must be made on an individual basis. Once dialysis is initiated for a patient with a chronic condition, it is continued for life or until the patient receives a successful kidney transplant. Thus many factors besides the medical ones must be considered. The following are considerations which should be evaluated before initiating hemodialysis:

MEDICOPSYCHOLOGICAL FACTORS:
    age
    cardiovascular condition
    metabolic conditions
    psychiatric stability

SOCIOREHABILITATIVE FACTORS:
    capability of rehabilitation
    motivation to function in family and community

PERSONAL ADJUSTMENT FACTORS:
    necessity of role reversal
    disturbances in sexual adequacy
    increased demands on family
    economic problems

REQUIRED DIALYSIS TEAM FOR CHRONIC CONDITIONS:
nephrologist
nurse
social worker
dietician
psychiatrist/psychologist

Complications

As with any mechanical treatment, technical problems can endanger the patient's life. Among the more common technical problems that can develop are a coil leak, kinked or disconnected tubings, and blood clots in the coil. Pyrogenic reactions due to bacterial growth have been known to occur. Cultures of the equipment should be taken.

It is vital to keep the blood from clotting in the coil. Two methods may be used. The systemic method is by direct intravenous injections of heparin into the patient. The dosage is determined by the clotting time within the coil, which must be carefully monitored. The second anticlotting method is regional. A heparin solution is allowed to flow into the coil. Protamine sulfate solution neutralizes the blood as it is returning to the patient. This method is especially useful when the patient is in danger of hemorrhaging.

Table 21-1 lists the most common complications in extracorporeal hemodialysis, their causes, and their corrections.

TABLE 21-1. COMPLICATIONS DURING HEMODIALYSIS

Problem	Cause	Correction
Hypovolemia	ECF volume depletion	Administer NaCl; slow down machine.
Arterio-venous spasm or collapse	Machine operating too fast	Slow machine; apply warm moist packs; administer NaCl.
Hypotensive shock	Volume depletion or hemorrhage	Administer blood and/or NaCl.
Arrhythmias	Potassium excess or deficit	Derive treatment from serum potassium level and cardiac monitor readings.
Hemorrhage	Stress ulcer; systemic heparinization	Use regional heparinization; transfuse.
Disequilibrium syndrome	Overly rapid correction of severe uremia causing cerebral edema	Avoid abrupt reduction of BUN.
Air emboli	Dry fluid line; air in venous line	Do not allow fluid line to go dry.

Nurse's Responsibilities

The shunt is the patient's "life line" to the artificial kidney and requires special attention from the nurse. The nurse should observe for warmth and pulsation. Report a stringy appearance of the blood or suspicions of clotting to the physician at once. Prompt irrigation can often save the shunt. Clamps and a tourniquet should be readily available in case the shunt comes apart or comes out.

Problems which directly affect the shunt are coagulation defects, vascular problems usually due to thrombophlebitis or inadequate blood vessels, and hemorrhage.

Since the patient requiring extracorporeal hemodialysis will have many emotional difficulties along with his medical problems, the nurse should be available to provide emotional support as an integral part of good nursing care.

BIBLIOGRAPHY

Davidson, R. C., and Scribner, B. H.: A Physician's Syllabus for the Treatment of Chronic Uremia. University of Washington, Seattle, 1967.

Eschbach, J. W., et al.: Erythropoiesis in patients with renal failure undergoing chronic dialysis. N. Engl. J. Med. 276:653, 1967.

Hampers, C. L., et al.: Megaloblastic hematopoiesis in uremia and in patients on long-term hemodialysis. N. Engl. J. Med. 276:551, 1967.

Quinton, W., Dillard, D., and Scribner, B. H.: Cannulation of blood vessels for prolonged hemodialysis. Trans. Am. Soc. Artif. Intern. Organs 6:104, 1960.

NOTES

22

Gastrointestinal Intubation and Tube Feeding

Gastrointestinal intubation and tube feeding are pertinent to fluid and electrolyte balance because they either subtract from or add to the body's fluids and electrolytes. In either of these processes the electrolyte and acid-base balance may also be altered. Discussed here are the various types of gastrointestinal tubes, their indications, and methods of insertion.

Rubber or plastic tubes are inserted into the stomach through the nose or mouth, or through the abdomen into the stomach by a surgical technique called a gastrostomy. In a gastrostomy the tubing is held in place by sutures and a retention catheter. These techniques may be used for decompression, irrigation and cleansing, feeding, or aspiration of the contents of the stomach for tests.

When used for decompression, intubation relieves abdominal distress caused by lack of peristalsis, which sometimes follows surgery, or by reverse peristalsis, which sometimes accompanies an intestinal obstruction. Without adequate peristalsis, gaseous and liquid substances build up in the stomach and cause distress. Intestinal distress is discussed below.

Irrigation and cleansing (**lavage**) may be performed when a toxic substance has been introduced into the stomach. Irrigation is used to maintain the patency of the gastric tube.

The gastric tube may also be used to deposit nutrients directly into the stomach when the patient has difficulty ingesting food. Tube feedings administer calories, nutrients, and especially the protein necessary for tissue healing.

Conditions in which patients may require gastric tube feeding include disorientation, confusion, unconsciousness, mental illness, extreme weakness caused by chronic debilitating illnesses, difficulty in swallowing, severe anorexia, and oral surgery. Naturally, feeding by intubation is not a preferred method, but it is sometimes necessary to maintain the patient's nutritional state until other problems can be improved or remedied.

GASTRIC INTUBATION

Types of Gastric Tubes

The most common and familiar gastric tube, the Levin tube, is a single lumen rubber or plastic tube. In adult sizes, it usually ranges from 12 to 18

French units. The tube should be 12 to 24 inches longer than the length from the patient's mouth to his stomach.

Some newer types of nasogastric tubes are made of radiopaque substances to facilitate the examination of placement by X ray.

Other types of gastric tubes have a sump airway that partially suspends the tube to keep it from coming in close contact with the gastric mucosa. The sump thus enhances the collection of specimens and suction, as the tube does not become occluded as easily. It also prevents damage to the gastric mucosa, especially during suctioning.

Insertion Procedure

The patient should be physically and psychologically prepared for the insertion of a gastric tube. Prior to insertion, rubber tubes are chilled in ice to stiffen them, thereby enhancing easy passage. Chilling also reduces friction and lessens irritation to the mucosa during insertion. Plastic tubes are firmer than rubber tubes, and do not need to be chilled; in fact, they may need to be warmed if they are too firm. The plastic tube becomes more pliable once it is inserted, and it will then conform to the anatomy. Allow six to eight inches of the tube to hang freely in order to determine the natural curve of the tube. Follow the natural curve of the tube to aid the ease of insertion. Use a water soluble lubricant. An oil base lubricant is more likely to incite pneumonitis if it is aspirated.

The gastric tube may be inserted through the nares or the oral cavity to the stomach. A nasal insertion is usually preferred over an oral insertion, because it is less likely to stimulate the gag reflex. Nasogastric insertion is usually used if the tube is to be left in place over a long period. The orogastric approach is used when the nares are structurally abnormal or when intubation will be used only for a short time. Nasogastric insertion is also contraindicated in the presence of nasal trauma with bleeding or when the tube is too large to pass through the nares. Orogastric intubation is also used when the patient prefers it.

Nasogastric Insertion

If possible, the patient should be in an upright position. If the patient must remain supine, position him on his right side. These positions facilitate the gravity passage of the tube.

Explain the procedure to the patient as it is performed. The patient's cooperation will make passage of the tube easier.

Determine the length of tubing needed prior to insertion by measuring from the tip of the patient's nose to the ear lobe and from the ear lobe to the end of the sternum. The average measurement for an adult is from 18 to 22 inches. This measurement is an estimate of the length of tube needed to reach the stomach. Prior to insertion, mark the measurements or use the scale marked on the tube, counting from the end of the tube to the desired length. When the tube has been inserted as far as the nose to ear lobe measurement, ask the patient to begin swallowing to assist the passage of the tube into the esophagus.

Lubricate the tube well with water-soluble jelly unless specimens for cytology are to be obtained. Lubricant will interfere with the visibility of the cells. Jelly, water, or saline can be used for lubrication. Water soluble material should be used in case the tube enters the trachea. Grease jellies are irritating to the respiratory tract and may cause a pneumonitis.

To insert the tube into the nostril, grasp the tube about three inches from the lubricated end. Holding the tube close to the end makes the tube stiffer and facilitates entry. Hold the nares upward and advance the tube forward and downward. The upward position of the nares straightens the passageway which the tube must follow. Do not force the tube if there is resistance. Using force could cause trauma to the mucosa and break the blood vessels. If no resistance is felt, pass the tube to the back of the oropharynx which should be about the premeasured distance from the tip of the nose to the ear lobe. The patient's eyes may tear as passage of the tube stimulates the tear glands and ducts.

Ask the patient to flex his head until his chin rests on his chest. This position will encourage the tube to enter the posterior pharynx and then the esophagus. The patient should now begin swallowing; remind him not to breathe deeply. Swallowing helps move the tube into the esophagus rather than the trachea. Deep breathing, on the other hand, tends to draw the tube into the trachea. At this point, ask the patient to open his mouth and determine whether or not the tube is circling in the mouth. Peristalsis of the esophagus also helps advance the tube. If the patient is unable to swallow, stroke his throat upward, toward the chin. The stroking causes swallowing which closes the epiglottis and increases pharyngeal contraction and esophageal peristalsis.

If excessive coughing, cyanosis, or inability to speak occur, withdraw the tube. These are signs that the tube has passed into the larynx and is stimulating the cough reflex in the trachea.

Since advancement of the tube often stimulates the gag reflex, it may be necessary to stop advancement for a short time until gagging is controlled. Instruct the patient to pant until the gagging sensation passes. Panting helps decrease the psychological aspects of gagging.

Do not advance the tube if resistance is encountered. Resistance may indicate the presence of an obstruction or abnormality. Report this to the physician.

When the premeasured length has been inserted, check the placement of the tube. If a radiopaque tube has been used, X ray is the most accurate means of evaluating tube placement. Radiopaque tubes, however, are not commonly used. A second method of checking the placement is to aspirate gastric contents with an asepto bulb or syringe. A return of gastric secretions means that the tube is in the stomach. No secretions returned does not mean the tube is not in the stomach; however, in this case, tube placement must be verified by some other method. Shifting the patient's position so he is lying on his left side will sometimes result in a return of gastric secretions. A third method of verification involves placing the distal end of the tube in a glass of water. If the tube is in the stomach, there may be limited erratic bubbling. If the bubbling is regular and coincides with the patient's respiration, the tube is probably in the trachea. A fourth method of verifying the tube's position is by injecting about five cc of air into the tube with a syringe while using a stethoscope to listen for a "swooshing" sound as the air enters the stomach. Do not instill any liquids into the tube until the position of the tube has been verified. If the tube is in the trachea, administration of liquids could suffocate the patient.

Secure the gastric tube by taping it to the nose and/or cheek. A good taping method is to split a two to three inch long tape about half way down, leaving two tails. Affix the unsplit portion of the tape to the nose, and wrap the two tails around the tube. This method of taping prevents the tube from jiggling, which could stimulate the gag reflex or irritate the nares. Do not tape the tube tightly against the nares opening because a pressure sore can develop.

Depending on the use of the tube, either attach the tube to suction or clamp the tube by doubling it back on itself. If suction is indicated, set the siphonage on a low pressure setting. High pressure may traumatize the gastric mucosa. While the tube is being prepared, ready the suction machine by turning it on and clamping the connecting tubing, allowing suction to build up.

Proper oral care is extremely important during intubation. The tube stimulates the mucosa and can become an irritant. Patients with gastric tubes tend to mouth-breathe, which dries the membranes. Application of a lemon and glycerin mixture will decrease both of these annoyances. Because there is no food to stimulate the salivary glands, they may not empty and **parotitis** may develop. Sucking on hard, sour candy may eliminate this problem. However, this may be contraindicated since it will also stimulate the gastric juices which may promote ulcer formation. Excessive gagging may also be a problem for some patients. Gagging can be controlled to some degree by administering an antacid to coat the pharynx. If this is ineffective, an anesthetic agent which decreases the sensations of the pharynx may be used. Anesthetics commonly used for this purpose are lidocaine spray, lidocaine viscous, and Cetacain. A mouthwash should be made available to the patient to alleviate some of the bad tastes and odors which accompany intubation.

Orogastric Insertion

Oral insertion of a gastric tube follows the same basic principles as nasal insertion. The variations in the procedure needed for oral insertion follow.

To premeasure the length of the tubing needed to reach the stomach, measure from the lips to the base of the sternum. Place the tube over the center and toward the back of the patient's tongue. The tube is thereby inserted into the posterior pharynx area.

Ask the patient to suck on the tube as if it were a straw and, at the same time, to swallow. The contractions of the pharynx will pull the tube backward. Stimulation of the gag reflex may be decreased if, after inserting the tube about six inches, the tube is moved to the left cheek area between the teeth and the cheek.

Advance the tube the required distance. Check the placement of the tube by one of the four methods previously described. Secure the tube to the cheek and either clamp it or connect it to the suction.

Removal of Gastric Tube   Clamp the end of the tube to prevent gastric secretions from dropping into the trachea. Remove the tape securing the tube.

Instruct the patient to inhale deeply and then to exhale slowly while the tube is being removed. This facilitates removal of the tube and prevents aspiration of gastric secretions into the trachea. The tube should be pulled out in one continuous motion.

Because many patients are nauseated by the sight of the tube, wrap it in a towel as it is removed. Assist the patient with oral care to prevent irritation and nausea due to the tube. Clean or dispose of the tube as indicated by institutional policy.

TUBE FEEDING

Gastric **gavage,** the introduction of nutrients into the stomach by mechanical means, is another term used for tube feeding. Gavage is indicated when the patient is unable to maintain adequate nourishment by other means, but still has patent gastric and intestinal passageways and normal digestion patterns. The physician will prescribe the amount, frequency, and kind of feeding as he would for any other diet. Tube feedings are usually prepared in liquid form in a blender and stored in the refrigerator on the unit.

The caloric requirements are based on the patient's weight and body needs. Calories are administered primarily for their protein-sparing action. If the protein supply is not adequate, the body cannot make and repair tissues and may eventually burn body proteins for energy. Nutrients burned for energy are consumed in the following order: carbohydrates, then fats, and then proteins. The nurse should be alert to inadequate intake and utilization and correct these by whatever method will improve the patient's nutritional status.

Methods

There are basically three methods of tube feedings, the difference being in the type of equipment used. One method utilizes an asepto or calibrated syringe, another the drip-regulated bag, and the third a food pump, such as the Barron food pump. All accomplish the same task, but with selective differences.

Asepto Syringe Methods. A Levin tube or a gastrostomy tube is inserted while the patient is in a semi-Fowler's position. Measure the amount of tube feeding ordered in a graduated cylinder and warm to room temperature. The warming of the liquid should be carefully controlled, since most of the liquids used for tube feedings are an excellent medium for bacterial growth.

Check the placement of the Levin tube to insure that it is in the stomach. Pour the feeding into the asepto or other syringe attached to the tube. A catheter adaptor is needed to fit the syringe to the Levin tube; the asepto will fit naturally without leaking. Gravity flow is the most common means for the passage of the liquid through the tube. The rate of flow is controlled by the height at which the asepto is placed. If the solution does not flow easily, the feeding may need to be thinned. Check the physician's orders before thinning it. In some cases, the flow can be started by applying a small amount of pressure by using the bulb of the asepto syringe or plunger. Avoid rapid administration, since it tends to increase gastric discomfort and to stimulate the gastrocolic reflex. Feedings high in calories may precipitate diarrhea. Some tube feedings are colored, usually blue, to detect fistulae. At no time should air be allowed to enter the tubing.

Approximately 30 minutes are required for a 200 to 300 cc fluid feeding. After completion of the feeding, the tubing should be rinsed with 50 to 75 cc of water. This may be specified by the physician. The water need not be sterile. The amount of water may need to be adjusted according to the fluid needs of the patient, as well as to the amount of rinsing needed to prevent agglutination of the fluid in the tube.

Fold the tube back on itself, then double clamp the tube to prevent leaking.

Drip-Regulated Method. The basic principles of the asepto syringe method are also applicable to the drip-regulated method. Therefore, only the variations in the method are discussed here.

A graduated measure bag attached to a drip chamber administers the feeding gradually at a prescribed rate. The flow is regulated by adjustment of the clamp and the height of the bag. Rinse the Levin tubing by flushing with water after the feeding.

Mechanical Food Pump Method. The food pump method differs from the previous methods in that the nutrients are actually pumped by an electric machine under pressure into the stomach. The Levin or gastrostomy tube is inserted as previously described. Unlike the other methods, the mechanical food pump maintains a continuous flow of nutrients at a constant rate. The other methods do not provide this accuracy in maintaining a constant flow. The asepto method feeding is of short duration; the rate of flow is adjusted by the height of the asepto bag. The drip-regulated method more closely resembles the mechanical food pump in that nutrients are administered continuously over a longer period of time. However, the rate of flow from this apparatus is also determined by the height of the container and the tension of the clamp. Moreover, in feedings of longer duration, the fluid cannot be iced as it hangs in the bag from a standard. Thus the food pump is preferred for more continuous, slowly administered tube feedings. The food is in a graduated, closed container that can be kept in an ice chest to keep the food from spoiling as it is administered.

The food pump connective tubing is attached to the gastric tube by a glass or plastic connector. Pulleys, usually on the underside of the pump, control the rate of flow, which is regulated in terms of cc/hour. Figure 22-1 shows the pulley system of a food pump. This particular machine has four rates; very slow (43 cc/hr), slow (65 cc/hr), moderate (113 cc/hr), and fast (200 cc/hr). The rate is determined by the feeding volume and the time period specified by the physician. Because continuous feeding is required, the liquid should never be allowed to clog up in the tubing. If the feeding is thick and to be given slowly, it may be necessary to periodically administer some water to rinse the tubing. A close tabulation of quantity and type of intake should be kept. Even the patient receiving substantial amounts of nutrients needs some additional water intake.

As the fluid container gradually empties, the end of the tubing must be kept below the level of the fluid so that air is not pumped into the stomach, causing distention.

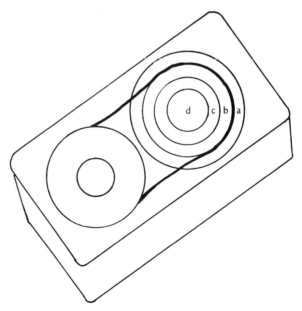

Figure 22-1. Pulley system of food pump-administration rate: a) very slow; b) slow; c) moderate; d) fast.

During continuous feedings, the patient must be monitored to be sure that the feeding is not being administered too rapidly. Rapid feeding may incite nausea and vomiting from the high caloric intake or distention which may cause spasms of the diaphragm exhibited by hiccoughs **(singultus)**. Slowing the feeding down or discontinuing it for a short time will aid the patient.

It is advisable to keep the upper trunk and head of the tube-fed patient slightly elevated to avoid aspiration if the patient vomits. Sometimes turning the patient on his side is helpful. If the patient is on a respirator or has a cuffed endotracheal or tracheotomy tube, the cuff should be kept inflated to prevent the possibility of aspiration during vomiting. The cuff should be inflated approximately thirty minutes to one hour after the feeding.

INTESTINAL INTUBATION

Intestinal tubes are most commonly used for decompression of the intestinal tract or as a presurgical aid. Decompression is the removal of both gaseous and liquid substances from the intestines. This relieves the pressure in the intestines caused by flatus. Flatus or gas is usually due to slowed or absent peristalsis caused by anesthesia or by surgery in which the intestines have been manipulated. Peristalsis may also be upset by an intestinal obstruction which may actually cause the intestines to contract in a reverse direction in an attempt to move the secretions out of the body. This is the reason that nausea and vomiting, possibly projectile, are often seen in the patient with an intestinal obstruction.

The most commonly used intestinal tubes are the Miller-Abbott and the Cantor tubes. The Miller-Abbott tube is a double lumen tube usually made of rubber. It is ten feet long and most frequently 16 French in diameter. The lumens are independent of each other. One lumen is used for inflation of the bulb at the end of the tube. The balloon and metal tip assist forward movement. The other lumen is for the aspiration of gas and secretions and is connected to a thermotic type of suction which pulls the gas and secretions out by vacuum.

Before the tube is inserted, it should be stiffened by chilling. The physician usually inserts the tube, frequently through the nose into the stomach in the same manner as the Levin tube. Before insertion, the tube must be measured for the correct length. The markings on the tube can be used for an estimate.

The tube is *not* taped to the nose after insertion. The tube must be free so that the action of peristalsis can draw it into the intestines. If the tube were anchored, it could not move into place in the duodenum. The tube may be coiled and placed in a plastic sack attached to the patient's gown. This will enable the tube to move and will keep the patient from becoming entangled in the tubing. Varying the position of the patient often aids the movement of the Miller-Abbott tube. Allowing a time lapse between each shift, turn the patient first to his right side, then to his back, and then to his left side. X ray will verify the placement of the tube.

The progress of advancement can be monitored by checking the scale marked on the tube. The physician may order the nurse manually to advance the tube into the stomach, designating the times and distances of the advancement.

The Cantor tube is a ten foot, single lumen tube. An 18 French diameter is most commonly used. Its main characteristic is a mercury-filled bag at the end of the rubber tubing to facilitate gravity flow insertion. The physician will insert a specific amount of mercury (usually 5 cc) into the bag with a needle and syringe. Because of its density, the mercury will not leak out of the rubber bag. As with the Miller-Abbott tube, the physician is usually responsible for insertion. Advancement of the tube may be ordered. The physician may choose to advance the tube under fluoroscopy to allow him to observe the movement of the tube by X ray.

Nursing service policy will determine whether removal of the tube is the responsibility of the physician or the nurse. It is often the physician's responsibility.

Nurse's Responsibilities

Prepare the patient for the intubation procedure.

Maintain accurate intake and output records.

Irrigate tubes with normal saline.

Observe for fluid and electrolyte imbalances due to losses from suctioning (extracellular fluid deficit, hypokalemia, acidosis [intestinal intubation], alkalosis [gastric intubation]).

Provide oral and nasal care.

Provide emotional support and physical comfort.

BIBLIOGRAPHY

Brunner, L., et al.: Textbook of Medical-Surgical Nursing, ed. 3. J. B. Lippincott Company, Philadelphia, 1975.

Burrell, L. O., and Burrell, Z. L., Jr.: Intensive Nursing Care. The C. V. Mosby Company, St. Louis, 1969.

Davol Rubber Company: Instructions for the Use and Assembly of Davol Miller-Abbott Tube. Providence, Rhode Island, 1969.

Dison, N. G.: An Atlas of Nursing Techniques, ed. 2. The C. V. Mosby Company, St. Louis, 1971.

Metheny, N. M., and Snively, W. D., Jr.: Nurses' Handbook of Fluid Balance, ed. 2. J. B. Lippincott Company, Philadelphia, 1974.

Moss, G.: Iced saline lavage for stomach hemorrhage. RN 35:icu 1-2, 1972.

Priestly, J. W.: A nurse's role in a gastro-enterology investigation unit. Nurs. Times 68:47, 1972.

Roche Handbook of Differential Diagnosis. Hoffmann-La Roche, Inc., Nutley, New Jersey, 1969.

Sutton, A. L.: Bedside Nursing Techniques in Medicine and Surgery. W. B. Saunders Company, Philadelphia, 1964.

Wintrobe, M., et al. (eds.): Harrison's Principles of Internal Medicine, ed. 6. McGraw-Hill, New York, 1970.

NOTES

NOTES

23

Venipuncture

Intravenous therapy is the practice of administering fluids, nutrients, or drugs directly into the bloodstream through a venous opening called a venipuncture. As with gastrointestinal intubation and tube feeding, intravenous therapy influences fluid and electrolyte balance.

Intravenous therapy has several purposes. It may be used to replace fluids and nutrients more rapidly than by oral administration. It is also used to sustain patients who are unable to take substances orally. Another important use is to administer drugs that must be instantly available to the body, such as those administered to patients with arrhythmias.

Patient Preparation

Successful intravenous therapy depends, in part, on preparing the patient both psychologically and physically. The nurse's approach is very important. If the nurse acts suddenly and sternly, the patient may infer that his condition has deteriorated. Seeing intravenous equipment may imply a crisis situation to the patient and his family, since people often associate intravenous therapy with critical and potentially death-producing situations. Thus it is imperative to prepare the patient by explaining both the procedure of venipuncture and the purpose of intravenous therapy in terminology which is both appropriate and understandable to each particular patient and his family.

Selection of Intravenous Fluids

It is important for the nurse to be familiar with the types of fluids (solutions) utilized and procedures for their safe administration. Before its administration, intravenous fluid should be checked against the physician's orders for type, amount, per cent of solution, and rate of flow. The nurse should be aware of situations that contraindicate particular solutions. For example, a patient with congestive heart failure should usually not be given a saline solution because this type of fluid encourages the retention of water, and would therefore augment the pump failure by increasing the fluid overload. Close evaluation of the type of fluid administered is also required for patients with renal and liver diseases, the elderly, and the very young, as these groups of people cannot tolerate an excessive fluid volume.

217

Selection of Site

When selecting a venipuncture site, consider these factors: the characteristics of the site, the purpose and duration of the infusion, the kind and amount of fluid administered, the condition of the vein, and the patient's overall comfort and condition.

The available sites are the superficial veins of the extremities. The most commonly used veins in the order of the frequency of their use are as follows:

1. veins of the forearm (basilic, cephalic)
2. veins around the **cubital fossa** (antecubital, cephalic, basilic)
3. veins in the radial area
4. veins in the hand
5. veins in the thigh (femoral, saphenous)
6. veins in the foot
7. veins in the scalp (infant and elderly).

(See Figures 23-1 through 23-3.)

The most frequently used sites are the veins of the forearm. The veins of both arms should be inspected very closely before selecting a site. If possible, do not use the patient's dominant arm since venipuncture restricts movement.

Leg veins are not usually used by the nursing staff for venipuncture because of the danger of **phlebothrombosis** and thrombophlebitis, which are greater in the legs than in the arms. Thrombophlebitis can lead to the release of emboli that can lodge in the lungs.

The most accessible vein is not necessarily the most ideal site. The antecubital space, for example, has a large vein more easily accessible than a distal location. However, use of the antecubital area restricts movement of the arm. Bending the elbow may easily obstruct the flow of solution, causing infiltration which could lead to thrombophlebitis. If the area infiltrates, moreover, the lower veins cannot usually be used for further puncture sites. It is preferable to start the infusion *distally* to provide the option of proceeding up the extremity if the vein is ruptured or infiltrated.

In considering use of the fossa area, the close proximity of the artery to the vein should be noted in order to avoid puncturing it (see Figure 23-4). Acute, severe pain in the arm and hand upon venipuncture usually indicates an arteriospasm. Remove the needle and apply pressure for five minutes or until bleeding stops.

The size of the veins must be considered in relation to the amount and type of fluid to be administered and the duration of therapy. Veins in the back of the hand are small, roll more easily, and are often difficult to anchor. Thus forearm veins may be preferred for therapy of longer duration.

Thus, the purpose of the infusion influences the selection of a site. If the purpose is the replacement of blood, a large vein should be used because of the **tonicity** of the solution. The thicker solution requires a larger vein and needle caliber to sustain an adequate flow. The peripheral vascular pressure in the patient may be increased enough to make it difficult for the blood to flow freely into the vein. In fact, because of its viscosity, the blood may have to be mechanically pumped into the patient's vein. Infusion of large quantities requires a larger vessel.

When hypertonic or irritating solutions are to be administered, use of a larger vein should be considered. Both of these solutions produce an inflammatory reaction in the vessel causing some local edema that narrows the caliber of the vessel. There may not be a sufficient blood flow in the smaller veins to dilute the tonicity of the solution, and further irritation may develop.

The duration of therapy is another factor influencing the selection of the site. Larger vessels should be used when prolonged therapy is anticipated. The preservation of veins becomes critical during a prolonged course of intravenous therapy. Thus it is important to perform the initial venipuncture distally, performing each succeeding venipuncture more proximally. Using alternate arms for infusion will also help to preserve the veins.

The condition of the vein must be evaluated. A vein that is reddened or tortuous, or that rolls may not be a good site. In the aged, for example, the veins of the hand often roll and are surrounded by such thin skin that blood

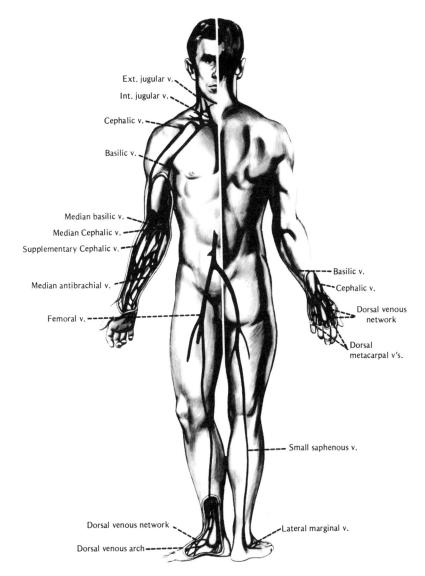

Figure 23-1.   Anterior and posterior superficial veins used for rapid injection of drugs and intravenous infusion of blood or fluids.*

*Figures 23-1 through 23-4 reprinted by permission from Venipuncture and Venous Cannulation, Abbott Laboratories, 1971.

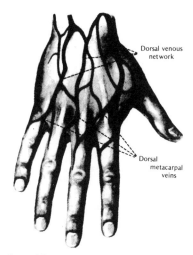

Figure 23-2.   Several suitable sites for venipuncture on the back of the hand.

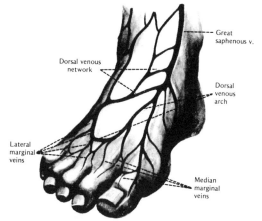

Figure 23-3.   Accessible venipuncture sites in the area of the foot.

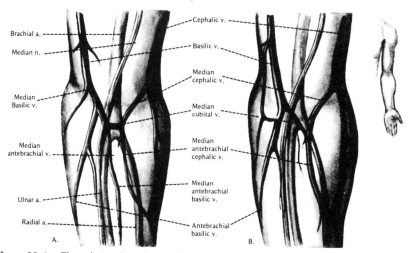

Figure 23-4.   The relationship of superficial arteries and nerves illustrated by two common vein arrangements of the antecubital fossa of the left arm.

can easily bleed into the interstitial spaces. If the patient is hypovolemic, the peripheral veins have a greater tendency to collapse than the proximal veins.

A thrombosed vein can be detected by palpation. It will feel hard and cord-like to the touch. Use of a thrombosed vein only increases the possibility of thrombophlebitis. Stagnation of blood, as in varicose veins, with the added trauma of venipuncture, also enhances the possibility of thrombophlebitis.

Edema in a potential site may make it difficult to locate the vein. Applying pressure in the local area may force the edema from the adjacent interstitial spaces and allow the vein to be palpated.

The consistent use of the same fingers for palpation will increase the nurse's sensitivity. Light pressure is recommended over heavy pressure for palpation of smaller peripheral vessels.

In summary, in the selection of a vein for venipuncture, the nurse must evaluate the characteristics of the site, the purpose and duration of the infusion, the kind and amount of fluid administered, and the condition of the vein.

Selection of Equipment

Since infusion equipment varies among companies, it is necessary to become familiar with the equipment available at the specific institution. However, there are some basic choices to make among the various types of equipment.

Needle Selection

Both metal and plastic needles or catheters are available for venipuncture.

Metal Needles. There are two types of metal needles: straight and scalp vein (intermittent) needles. The gauge of straight needles ranges from approximately 18 to 25. The smaller the gauge number, the larger the outside diameter of the needle. The scalp vein needle has an advantage over the straight needle in that it has a thinner wall allowing entry into a smaller vein. The shorter bevel of the scalp vein needle also reduces the chance of puncturing the wall of the vein opposite the point of entry. Plastic "butterfly" wings make it easier to hold the scalp needles for venipuncture.

In selecting metal needles, the gauge, the length of the needle, and the length of bevel should be considered. The gauge size will be determined by the amount, concentration, and duration of therapy. Moreover, the larger the quantity and the longer the duration of the *previous* infusion, the larger the subsequent gauge will need to be. If an infusion of blood is anticipated to follow an intravenous fluid, a larger gauge needle, such as a number 18, should be used. The gauge of the needle should be smaller than the vein chosen to lessen the amount of trauma to the vein and to facilitate adequate dilution of the fluid. If the gauge of the needle closely approximates the size of the vein, the limited amount of dilution of the intravenous fluid while it is running increases the irritation to the vein.

The length of the needle affects the flow rate. The longer the shaft of the needle, other factors being equal, the slower the flow. Shorter shafts lessen the chance of infiltration due to a "moving" needle.

A shorter bevel lessens the chance of puncture of the wall of the vein opposite the venipuncture and decreases the fluid loss into the interstitial spaces because less bevel opening is exposed while entering the vein. A shorter bevel also causes less trauma to the inner lining of the vein during venipuncture and infusion.

Shorter infusions are usually given with metal needles. Common sizes used are gauges of 20, 21, and 23 and lengths of one to one and one-half inches.

Plastic Needles. Plastic needles are often used for therapy of longer duration, usually extending from 12 to 24 hours. Plastic needles allow the patient more freedom of movement and cause less foreign body reaction. Care should be taken not to insert a plastic needle near a joint because flexion will obstruct the flow and may damage the needle.

There are three basic types of plastic needles. One type features a plastic catheter mounted on a metal needle. After venipuncture, the metal needle which was used to enter the vein is slipped out of the plastic catheter and removed. Intracatheter needles, the second type, have a catheter inserted through a metal needle, which is used only for the venipuncture and then removed. The third type is an inlying catheter that must be placed by a cut-down procedure involving a surgical incision by the physician. The vein is opened, and the catheter is secured in the vein by sutures.

Other Equipment

Other necessary equipment includes tubing, controlled volume sets, filters, and supportive equipment such as tourniquets or blood pressure cuffs, tape, armboards, and gauze.

The basic administration set includes tubing, a section for inserting the tubing into the bottle, and an adapter for connecting the tubing to the needle. (See Figure 23-5.) Note that this type of set contains only a drip chamber without a filter.

Controlled volume sets include tubing that regulates the size of drop or the amount that can be infused at one time. This includes the mini-drip, micro-drip, and volume chambers. The smaller drop size may be preferable to facilitate counting drops when slow drip rates are ordered. This is particularly true in administering intravenous fluids to infants or patients on restricted

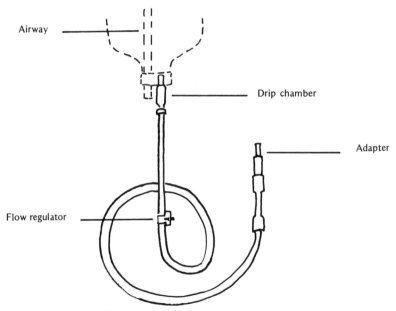

Figure 23-5.   Basic administration set.

fluid intake. Cardiac patients on a keep-open rate (KVO) and patients with renal or liver failure, for example, require close intravenous fluid monitoring. The volume chamber assures that only a minimum amount of fluid can be administered. This protects the patient from receiving the entire infusion in the case of a malfunction which suddenly increases the flow.

The use of filters is increasing. They are particularly useful in eliminating microscopic particles. The incidence of thrombophlebitis is now greatly reduced through the use of filters.

Tourniquets of various types and lengths may be used. A soft flexible band, similar to a one inch Penrose, is most common. The use of the sphygmomanometer is superior to the rubber tourniquet because the amount of pressure applied can be measured. Since the usual diastolic pressure is 80 mmHg, a pressure of 100 mm should be sufficient to increase engorgement of the peripheral vessels. In approximately 60 to 90 seconds the veins should be amply distended. If the veins do not sufficiently distend, apply warm, moist packs. Heat, to be effective, should be applied 10 to 20 minutes prior to venipuncture. Other methods of distending the veins include placing the extremity in a dependent position or mildly slapping the area, although some sources do not recommend slapping because of potential trauma. Having the patient open and close his fist may also help, as this muscular action forces more blood into the vein.

Procedure for Venipuncture

Prepare the patient psychologically and physically.

Prepare as much of the equipment as possible outside the room: Open the intravenous solution, connect the tubing, and select the needle. The drip chamber should be approximately one-third filled and the tubing cleared of air.

Proper lighting will aid venipuncture procedure.

Place the patient's arm on a firm surface in as comfortable a position as possible. If the arm is very hairy, shaving may be necessary.

Locate the vein by sight and/or palpation. Observe and palpate for the distended vein after application of the tourniquet. Select a site which fits the requirements previously discussed.

Cleanse the site area with an antiseptic solution, using a circular motion and moving from the center outward. The solution may vary according to institution. Some institutions use alcohol or iodine solutions when intracatheters and plastic needles are used because of the duration of therapy.

Use thumb to keep the skin taut, stabilizing the vein and the soft tissue surrounding it. This will help prevent rolling of the vein in the subcutaneous tissue during the venipuncture. A right-handed person should hold the extremity with his left hand, with the thumb positioned about two inches below the selected site for venipuncture.

Place the needle at a 45 degree angle in line with the selected vein. Insertion at this angle decreases the chance of puncturing the opposite wall of the vein. Check to be sure any curve of the vein is more than the length of the needle beyond the point of entry. The needle should not penetrate the curve of the vein since this would obstruct the flow. Keeping the bevelled edge of the needle up during entry into the skin and vein also helps to prevent puncturing the opposite wall. Some sources recommend rotating the bevel downward after piercing the skin and anterior wall to further decrease the chance of puncturing the posterior wall of the vein. The needle must enter the vein below the point selected for infusion, the site of entry depending on the length of the needle. The most commonly used lengths are one to one and one-half inches.

The needle may be inserted by a direct or indirect method. In the direct method, the needle is positioned on the skin directly over the vein and quickly thrust through both the skin and vein. In the indirect method, the needle enters through the skin slightly to the side of the vein. It is then moved toward the vein for entry.

Observe for a blood return while puncturing the skin and vein. As soon as blood returns in the tubing, the needle may be gently threaded up the vein. This step must be performed carefully with the needle parallel to the vein to insure that the walls of the vein are not punctured, causing infiltration and hematoma.

After the blood returns, release the tourniquet and open the tubing clamp. Establish that the infusion is flowing freely without an infiltration before taping the needle and tubing. Signs of infiltration are stinging, swelling, and cessation of flow.

The needle should be taped flush with the skin. Avoid taping directly over the bevel part of the needle as this may obstruct the flow. A small piece of tape may be placed beneath the hub of the needle. Another piece of tape is placed over the needle near the hub. Loop the tubing and secure it with tape independently of the needle so that tension applied to the tubing will only disturb the taped loop and will not jar the needle. Indicate the size of needle and the date on the tape for further reference. It is recommended that needles not be left in the vein of a patient over 48 hours.

An armboard may be used to prevent undue motion of the needle and arm that can lead to infiltration or thrombophlebitis. It is particularly useful in restraining the movement of infant, elderly, confused or uncooperative patients. Armboards vary in length. Short ones can be used to immobilize the wrist, longer ones for the elbows. An armboard is usually not needed with the small scalp vein needle. Place the board so as to immobilize the joints below and above the venipuncture. Tape the board, like the tubing, independently of the needle. If further restraint of movement of the tube is needed to prevent the dislodging of the needle, the tube can be secured to the board instead of to the patient. Commercial disposable armboards, padded for patient comfort, are now available.

Lastly, the solution should be administered according to the proper drip rate. The tubing should be free, and the intravenous pole positioned so as not to be bumped or knocked down. As an additional safety precaution, position the intravenous fluid bottles on the hook most distant from the patient. For ease in monitoring, mark the time of the infusion on the bottle.

Make the patient as comfortable as possible and encourage him to call the nurse if he feels discomfort. Intravenous infusions should be monitored every 15 to 30 minutes to insure adequate drip rate and to prevent infiltration. Record the time, site, type, and amount of solution on the chart. The size and length of needles may need to be charted, according to institutional policy.

Methods of venipuncture may vary according to institution. This chapter has stressed basic practices.

BIBLIOGRAPHY

Abbott Laboratories: Fluid and Electrolytes: Some Practical Guides to Clinical Use. Abbott Laboratories, North Chicago, 1970.

Abbott Laboratories: Parenteral Administration. Abbott Laboratories, North Chicago, Illinois, 1969.

Adriani, J.: Venipuncture. Am. J. Nurs. 62:66, 1962.

Dison, N. G.: An Atlas of Nursing Techniques, ed. 2. The C. V. Mosby Company, St. Louis, 1971.

Metheny, N. M., and Snively, W. D., Jr.: Nurses' Handbook of Fluid Balance, ed. 2. J. B. Lippincott Company, Philadelphia, 1974.

Plumer, A. L.: Principles and Practice of Intravenous Therapy, ed. 2. Little, Brown and Company, Boston, 1975.

Pfizer Laboratories: Intravenous Techniques. Spectrum 9:2, 1965.

Rosenfeld, M. G. (ed.): Manual of Medical Therapeutics, ed. 20. Little, Brown and Company, Boston, 1971.

Scribner, B. H. and Burnell, J. M.: Teaching Syllabus for Course on Fluid and Electrolyte Balance, ed. 7. University of Washington, Seattle, 1969.

Sutton, A. L.: Bedside Nursing Techniques of Medicine and Surgery, ed. 2. W. B. Saunders Company, Philadelphia, 1969.

NOTES

24

Intravenous Therapy

Immediate alteration of the fluid and chemical balance of the body frequently is necessary in modern health care. Intravenous therapy is the procedure that provides this life-sustaining function. It is a parenteral process because it involves the administration of substances to the body by means other than the intestinal tract.

The main purpose of intravenous therapy is the administration of fluid and nutrients in order to maintain or correct homeostasis. In recent health care practice intravenous therapy has also come to provide a means of keeping a venipuncture open (KVO) for administration of drugs in an emergency.

MAINTENANCE THERAPY

Maintenance intravenous therapy is used to sustain normal balance. It can be used in the patient who is not yet in a state where body fluids or chemicals are depleted but shows signs or has the possibility of becoming so. Maintenance therapy can be ordered for the patient who is allowed nothing by mouth (NPO) by doctor's orders in preparation for surgery or to decrease gastrointestinal upsets. Maintenance therapy can be ordered to prevent metabolic disturbances which would occur without the consumption of normal daily amounts of fluids, electrolytes, organic nutrients, and vitamins. It is frequently prescribed for patients who are comatose or unable to move and, therefore, in danger of aspirating vomitus.

Many times maintenance intravenous therapy is needed for the patient who cannot tolerate oral ingestion of fluids or nutrients and refuses to eat or drink. This includes patients who exhibit the signs and symptoms of anorexia, nausea, and vomiting. In the category of voluntary NPO, there is the condition in which the patient's thirst center, as a result of aging, post-trauma, or post-stress, is not stimulated even though the patient may need fluids. Unconscious patients are also candidates for maintenance intravenous therapy since the body is unable to indicate via the thirst centers when a fluid shortage occurs.

Regardless of whether the refusal to eat or drink is iatrogenic or patient-initiated, the emphasis in maintenance therapy is to supplement the patient's intake in order to keep the body from being thrown into either a fluid or nutrient deficit.

227

Maintenance fluids are generally composed of saline or isotonic water. Normal daily amounts of carbohydrates, electrolytes, and vitamins are included in this solution. A typical example is 5 per cent dextrose in water, potassium chloride, and vitamins B and C.

REPLACEMENT THERAPY

Replacement intravenous therapy is required when the patient is experiencing a fluid and/or nutrient deficit. There are basically two situations in which replacement therapy is utilized: one is an emergency situation and the other is in a condition in which the gastrointestinal tract is intolerant to food and/or fluids.

Replacement therapy is classified by the four areas in which an imbalance can develop: fluids, electrolytes, acid-base balance, and organic nutrients. Replacement nutrients are defined as nourishing substances including carbohydrates, fats, proteins, alcohol, water, electrolytes, minerals, and vitamins.

Fluid Loss and Replacement

Two types of fluid loss can occur in the body; they are water and saline loss.

Water loss is due to increased insensible loss, decrease in thirst center response, and lack of available water. Such losses are replaced by water and dextrose solutions. There are other types of water and sugar solutions but the water and dextrose combination is the most common intravenous solution used as a water replacement. At no time is **distilled water** used as a fluid replacement.

Saline losses can occur from any of the body cavities or fistulae when pancreatic and intestinal secretions or bile are dumped into the gastrointestinal tract and eliminated. Both vomiting and diarrhea may cause saline loss. Gastrointestinal loss, and hence saline loss, can also be precipitated by failure to replace fluids when gastrointestinal tubes such as the Levin, Miller-Abbott, or Cantor tubes are in place. Fluid lost through use of gastrointestinal tubes should be replaced proportionately.

Saline replacement is available in isotonic, hypotonic, and hypertonic solutions. Normal saline or one that is isotonic to blood plasma is a 0.9 per cent solution. In other words, it contains 140 mEq/L of sodium and 100 mEq/L of chloride.

Hypotonic solutions are most frequently labeled as a fraction of normal saline, i.e., one-fifth normal saline, one-third normal saline, or one-half normal saline. It is extremely important to be aware of whether isotonic or hypotonic saline is being administered. Isotonic solutions can be administered at a faster rate because they are compatible with the plasma. In contrast, a rapid administration of hypotonic solution can further upset the fluid balance of the body and cause water to move into the red blood cells, which results in the rupturing of the red blood cells (hemolysis).

Hypertonic solutions, ranging from 1 per cent to 5 per cent above normal saline, are also available. They are administered only when there is a profound loss of saline. This is because of the danger of inducing water to move from the blood cells into the plasma, thus causing shrinkage of the red blood cells (crenation). Such a water movement would overload the circulatory system and encourage the body to go into fluid overload states such as congestive heart failure, pulmonary edema, or renal failure.

In situations involving saline loss the primary problem is a fluid loss; however, some electrolytes are depleted along with the saline. These electrolytes include sodium and chloride.

Sodium and chloride can be lost secondary to the disease process. Examples of such losses are diabetes mellitus complicated by coma and renal failure during the salt-losing stage. Excessive sodium and chloride losses could include sensible losses which are accelerated as a result of pyrexia, hyperventilation, or use of ventilators. Diaphoresis can also result in sodium and chloride loss whether it is related to a disease syndrome or stimulated by the sympathetic nervous system as a part of the stress response. Iatrogenic losses may be due to drugs such as diuretics. Drug-induced losses occur if replacement is not planned into the health care regimen. Another possibility for fluid and an accompanying electrolyte loss is through drainage of certain types of wounds. Replacement needs to be related to the amount of drainage lost, this assessed by weighing the dressings or calculating the amount of drainage by some other means.

These electrolyte losses should be replaced by one of the saline solutions listed previously, such as normal saline.

One of the most important electrolytes to observe for replacement is potassium because there are no storage depots for this mineral in the body. Potassium losses can basically be classified as nonrenal and renal. (See Chapter 5 for detailed list.) Nonrenal depletions involve gastrointestinal losses, fistulae, and, according to some sources, episodes of diaphoresis. Renal losses occur during polyuria secondary to a disease state, from diuretic therapy, and from both a normal response and over-response to a stress situation.

Potassium can be added to the intravenous therapy fluid. It is available in 20 and 40 mEq vials. Patients who are not on a cardiac monitor should not receive more than 40 mEq/L solution or 20 mEq per hour. Potassium is never given intravenously as a direct undiluted solution. If a more rapid potassium replacement is required, the patient should be placed on a cardiac monitor in order to observe for potassium-induced arrhythmias. Always check for sufficient renal output before administering potassium.

Calcium is another electrolyte which should be monitored. Because of the importance of calcium in maintaining normal neuromuscular function, replacement therapy should be initiated when a calcium deficit appears. As with potassium, calcium can be lost through nonrenal and renal avenues. In addition to actual losses of calcium from the body, calcium can shift in and out of the tissue, thus giving the appearance of a deficit without actually depleting the quantity of calcium in the body. Should a false deficit situation arise, it may be necessary to administer calcium regardless of the fact that no actual deficit exists in order to combat the tetany which results from the unavailability of the calcium. Since this situation usually correlates to an acidotic state the best approach is to correct the acidosis. Ringer's lactate as a main intravenous therapy fluid can correct the acidosis, particularly in the case of diabetic acidosis (See Chapter 8).

Any administration of calcium through intravenous therapy must be at the physiological level, i.e., 9 to 11 milligrams per cent (10 per cent calcium). The first dose should be administered by a physician and the patient should be checked for hypersensitivity before further administration. Baseline information should be reviewed to determine whether or not the patient is using a digitalis because calcium enhances the possibility of digitalis intoxication.

Acid-Base Loss

Replacement   Acid-base imbalances occur secondary to a disease process or as a result of an emergency situation. (See Chapter 9 for pathophysiology.) The health team first needs to determine if the acid-base imbalance is alkalosis or acidosis. The two choices then are the replacement of acid to correct alkalosis or the replacement of base to correct acidosis.

Tetany, twitching, hyperirritability, and hyperreflexia are symptoms of alkalosis. These symptoms will decrease as the alkalotic state is alleviated. Solutions such as sodium chloride neutralize the excess base present in alkalosis by combining chloride ions with excess hydrogen ions of the base. This action acidifies the blood plasma and returns the pH balance to normal. Potassium chloride and arginine chloride also serve as acidifying intravenous therapy fluids. Because of the possibility of administering too much acid and creating acidosis, when administering acidifying solutions it is important to evaluate the pH readings as they become available and to monitor the patient for a decrease in the symptomatology that correlated with the alkalotic state.

Acidosis is usually secondary to a disease process such as diabetes, emphysema, or pneumonia. In acute diseases such as pneumonia or atelectasis or in emergency situations, short periods (such as one to three minutes) of apnea can convert the body into a state of metabolic acidosis as well as respiratory acidosis. This dual problem is created by the lack of metabolic oxygen to metabolize carbohydrates and the respiratory retention of carbon dioxide. The base, bicarbonate, is used to correct both metabolic and respiratory acidosis. In emergency situations acidosis is corrected by the administration of one to three ampules of sodium bicarbonate either as a direct venipuncture or by push.

Organic Nutrient Loss and Replacement   Organic nutrients can be replaced through parenteral means also. Sugar and protein are the two most common nutrients replaced through intravenous therapy. Hypoglycemia is a state in which the sugar in the blood drops so low that the body is thrown into a tetanic convulsive state. Immediate sugar replacement is required for brain cell metabolism. The hypoglycemic state can be caused by various factors. One factor is the excessive secretion of insulin, which is called the "rebound phenomenon." The rebound phenomenon occurs when large amounts of sugar are ingested and the body over-interprets the quantity of sugar present in the body. This causes the pancreas to secrete too much insulin, which drives the sugar too rapidly out of the blood and into the cells, thus precipitating a hypoglycemic state. This condition exists in about 5 per cent of the population.

Hypoglycemia may also be due to a stress response in which inadequate sugar is being consumed in proportion to the amount being burned. The too-rapid burning of sugar does not allow the body time to convert the sugar to glycogen and store it; hence the blood sugar level drops. Research is being done in the area of hypoglycemia related to psychogenic disorders.

Treated and untreated diabetes can create a hypoglycemic condition. In treated diabetes the patient may be taking more insulin than is needed to control his hyperglycemic condition or he may not be consuming enough food to balance his insulin injection. The result is hypoglycemia. In this type of hypoglycemia the situation is acute. It should be corrected by administration of prescribed amounts of nutrients *and* insulin or hypoglycemic agents in order to reestablish the body's balance.

Protein replacement may be prescribed in the case of a severe protein deficit. Substantial protein may be lost secondary to a disease process via the kidneys; from extensive burns through both the kidneys and the tissues, or in a postoperative situation in which hyperalimentation is being utilized as a form of therapy for severe anemia.

Protein solutions which are available include fractionated albumin, globulin, and combinations of the two. A typical example of protein replacement fluid is Amigen.

Prior to the administration of protein the patient should be checked for protein sensitivity. The protein solution should be diluted unless there is the possibility of a fluid overload. The patient should be observed for complaints of headache, nausea, vomiting, urticaria, pruritus, or frank shock which is indicated by cold clammy skin, drop in blood pressure, and respiratory and cardiac arrest. Should a hypersensitive reaction be allowed to continue it could result in anaphylactic shock.

RATE OF ADMINISTRATION

The amount and rate of administration in intravenous therapy will be calculated by the physician. Calculation ratios used are based on the weight of the patient, the amount of fluid needed for replacement, and condition of the patient's heart, lungs, and kidneys. Intravenous fluids are usually ordered on a per hour basis and calculated on a per minute basis. The fluid can be prescribed to run at a regular flow rate or by microdrops or minidrops. Drops per minute are calculated on the basis of the time period over which the IV will be administered.

The most effective rate for each patient is determined by two factors: the patient and the mechanical process of intravenous therapy. Factors relating to the patient are

    age
    weight or body circumference
    physical condition
    disease, if any
    other medications being consumed
    size of the vessels available for starting the venipuncture
    tolerance of the patient to the prescribed rate

Mechanical factors relating to the intravenous technique are

    the size of the needle
    the type of tubing
    thickness or tonicity of the solution
    weight or hydrostatic pressure of the solution
    need for rapid replacement vs. slow replacement
    peripheral resistance or back pressure from the patient
    IV plugs caused by local inflammatory response, clots at the end of the
        needle, needle pressing on the wall of the vein, or selection of a vein
        that is too small.

In an acute situation immediate steps must be taken to initiate intravenous therapy. Considerations in planning fluid needs are vital signs and an accurate intake and output record. The recording of intake and output must be accurate. False information can be worse than no information because treatments based on faulty information could easily complicate the situation.

PLANNING DAILY INTRAVENOUS THERAPY

The daily intravenous therapy plan is individualized for each patient's weight, age, cardiovascular and renal status, and disease condition. The patient's accelerated or decelerated body metabolism, which affects the amount of fluid and electrolytes lost and needed, should also be considered. This consideration is in addition to basic maintenance metabolic needs required by the NPO patient.

Prior to establishing a daily intravenous therapy plan obtain a complete history. Pay particular attention to information concerning the cardiovascular, respiratory, renal, hepatic, and endocrine systems. Review with the patient disease processes that would be related to known fluid and electrolyte imbalances. A history of hypertension which could progress to congestive heart failure should be noted. A patient with a history of Cushing's disease or one who has been on steroids will need to be observed for congestive heart failure and saline excess. Patients with Cushing's disease tend to hold salt and lose potassium, thereby developing hypokalemia and alkalosis. Any episode which in the past has led to fluid and electrolyte imbalances should be recorded. How the patient has tolerated stress with disease should be noted in terms of total body system compensation.

It is crucial that an accurate description be obtained of any fluid losses the patient has experienced. The amount and frequency of urination should be recorded. The patient should be asked to estimate the size of stools in cups, pints, or quarts. These figures could then be converted to cubic centimeters for registration in the history.

The degree of fever and hyperpnea are also important because both abnormalities will increase what are normally insensible losses into sensible losses. A normal insensible fluid loss is 1000 cc. per day afebrile, but in the febrile situation this loss is compounded by an additional loss caused by the increased respiratory rates. The result is a substantial total body loss.

After completing the patient's history make a thorough assessment. This is necessary in determining intravenous therapy needs. Evaluate the neural system. This includes particularly evaluation for hyperreflexia or hyporeflexia, lethargy, irritability, tetany, tremors, parathesia, and seizures and convulsions. Observe the nose and throat for mucous membrane changes, congestion, and hyperemia that are related to upper respiratory infections and which may be aggravated into an excessive saline loss secondary to fever. Examine the vascular system for rate and regularity of rhythm. Record heart sounds. Check the respiratory system for rate and rhythm. Measure the amount of ventilation, paying particular attention to hyperventilation and hypoventilation. Examine the abdomen for pain or tenderness.

Analysis of neck veins is important as a part of both physical assessment and bedside observation. Central venous pressure can be determined by a neck vein study. While the patient contracts his anal muscles, observe the height of the column of blood in the carotid vein in relationship to the jawline. The base of the elevation should be at the base of the jaw. A hypovolemic condition usually exists if it is lower. The diameter of the vein is also indicative of central venous pressure. A bulging vein indicates hypervolemia. A flat neck vein indicates hypovolemia.

Chemical assessment may be ordered. Baseline data includes hemoglobin, hematocrit, complete blood count, and a serum electrolyte for sodium, chloride, potassium, and carbon dioxide. Urine studies may also be part of the laboratory evaluation. A basic urinalysis, which includes determination of specific gravity and dilution of the urine, should also be ordered.

ADMINISTRATION

Check the physician's prescription against the commercially prepared mixture. Using a sterile procedure, open the bottle and insert the tubing. Remove the air from the tubing with a gravity technique. Attach the correct needle. Check the physician's order for the rate and amount of flow. Check the patient's chart for allergies and contraindications. (See Chapter 23, page 204, for technique for starting a venipuncture.)

When rapid fluid replacement is used monitor the patient for signs of fluid overload such as pulmonary edema, elevated pulse, elevated diastolic and systolic blood pressure, dyspnea, orthopnea, shortness of breath, anxiety, restlessness, burning at the site of administration, bubbling or wheezing-wet respiratory sounds.

IVs which were started with intracatheters and which will be in place for over 24 hours may require additional attention. Application of dressings may be needed. Observe for indications of local inflammatory response such as excessive wetness around the needle, swelling, slowing of the rate of infusion, return of blood with back pressure into the IV tubing.

IVs left in place over 48 hours may require application of ointments such as Bacitracin by sterile technique on the butterfly dressing to decrease the chance of iatrogenic infection.

WITHDRAWAL FROM INTRAVENOUS THERAPY

The intravenous apparatus should be removed when the patient no longer needs emergency administration of medication, replacement solutions, or maintenance solutions. Homeostasis is now being maintained by adequate fluid intake. Establishment of adequate intake is determined prior to discontinuing the IV. It is important also to chart gastrointestinal tolerations of fluids and to be sure the pH balance has stabilized before removing the IV.

Sterile procedures for withdrawal should be utilized. The following procedures should be performed:

apply alcohol sponge with pressure on the needle site
turn off the IV
quickly withdraw the needle from the site in the same angle at which it
    was originally inserted
apply pressure to the site for a minimum of 3 minutes to prevent blood
    leakage into the tissue, which would result in ecchymosis
cover the opening with a sterile dressing or tape.

Measures in post-intravenous therapy include observation for homeostatic return of all fluids and electrolytes, observation of acid-base balance and nutrient balance, and observation of cardiac, respiratory, and renal functions. Check foods and fluids for gastrointestinal tolerance and record intake and output.

BIBLIOGRAPHY

Brooks, D. K., et al.: Osmolar and electrolyte changes in haemorrhagic shock. Hypertonic solutions in the prevention of tissue damage. Lancet 1:521, 1963.

Burke, S. R.: Composition and Function of Body Fluids, ed. 2. C. V. Mosby Company, St. Louis, 1976.

Goldberger, E.: The Treatment of Cardiac Emergencies. C. V. Mosby Company, St. Louis, 1974.

Parenteral Administration. Abbott Laboratories, North Chicago, Illinois, 1969.

Plumer, A. L.: Principles and Practice of Intravenous Therapy, ed. 2. Little, Brown and Company, Boston, 1975.

Smith, J.: Manual of Medical Therapeutics, ed. 19. Little, Brown and Company, Boston, 1969.

Stephenson, H. E., Jr.: Immediate Care of the Acutely Ill and Injured. C. V. Mosby Company, St. Louis, 1974.

Weldy, N. J.: Body Fluids and Electrolytes: A Programmed Presentation. C. V. Mosby Company, St. Louis, 1976.

NOTES

236

25

Tracheotomy Care

Tracheotomy is a surgical procedure that makes an artificial opening into the "windpipe" or trachea for the insertion of a tube. Tracheotomy is performed to alleviate airway problems. This chapter is included because any variation in the respiratory pattern may affect the acid-base balance. The reasons for tracheotomy and the care of the patient that has one are discussed.

The term tracheotomy usually refers to a temporary opening, while tracheostomy usually refers to a permanent opening. These terms, however, are often used interchangeably. A temporary opening is generally used in an emergency situation until normal ventilation can be established; a permanent opening is used when there is no chance of the patient regaining a normal airway.

The trachea is composed of C-shaped rings of cartilage which begin just below the larynx. In a tracheotomy, the opening is usually made into the trachea at the level of the third or fourth ring. If the opening is made above the level of the second ring, surgical complications may result from injury to the larynx, nerve damage, and hemorrhage. Fortunately, these complications seldom occur.

Indications for Tracheotomy

There are two categories of patients requiring tracheotomy: those with an airway obstruction and those with a medical problem requiring improved air intake. Examples of airway obstructions include tumors, foreign bodies, edema of the larynx, severe infections of the neck, larynx, or oral cavity, trauma, and mucus plugs. In any airway obstruction, a danger of asphyxia exists. Signs and symptoms that indicate the imminence of asphyxia are dyspnea, **inspiratory stridor** (a harsh, high-pitched sound), **sternal retraction,** and restlessness. The skin color changes from pale to pallor and cyanosis. Remember that cyanosis is a late sign.

The second category of patients includes those who cannot expectorate their secretions or those who need to increase their tidal volume by decreasing the amount of air in the dead space. For example, in the case of chronic obstructive pulmonary disease, a tracheotomy is performed to diminish the amount of dead space that exists from the mouth to the sternal region,*

---

*Sigmund Grollman: The Human Body, Its Structure and Physiology. Collier Macmillan Limited, London, 1969, p. 287.

thereby supplying extra oxygenated air. Other examples of patients in this category include those with head injury and unconsciousness, those with musculoskeletal diseases, and those with fractured ribs, who are unable to cough because of the pain. The major goals of tracheotomy are to increase the efficiency of ventilation and to minimize the work of breathing.

Laboratory Tests. Laboratory tests may indicate the need for better ventilation. Progressive hypercapnia (increased pCO_2), hypoxemia (decreased pO_2), and acidosis (decreased pH) may be present. The degree of hypoxia precipitates observable changes in the respiratory pattern: initially the respiratory center is stimulated; as the obstruction continues, the center is depressed.

Normal tidal volume is 500 to 600 cc per respiration. Of this, 150 cc (or 1 cc/1 lb. body weight) occupies the dead space, so that the patient is actually utilizing 350 to 450 cc of oxygenated air with each respiration. The functional tidal volume inhaled by the patient will increase with the elimination of some of the dead space through the insertion of a tracheotomy tube.

Types of Tracheotomy Tubes

Tracheotomy tubes are made of silver, plastic, or rubber. They may have a single or double cuff or no cuff. Children's sizes range from 00 to 3 with a 65° angle. Adult sizes range from 3 to 8, with a 90° angle. The most frequently used adult sizes are from 4 to 6. The tube used for a **laryngectomy** will be larger, usually in the range of 8 to 9, to keep the stoma dilated. A basic tracheotomy set consists of an outer cannula, an inner cannula, and an obturator (see Figure 25-1). Some of the newer rubber and plastic sets contain only an outer cannula and obturator.

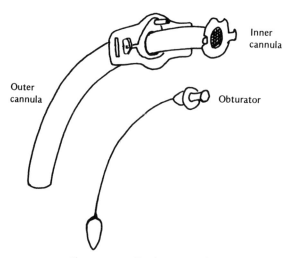

Figure 25-1.   Tracheotomy tube.

Tracheotomy Care

The patient and his family must be prepared for the tracheotomy prior to surgery. The resultant edema and the need to learn to redirect air after surgery will cause the patient temporary difficulty in talking. Therefore, the patient and his family should be familiarized with alternative means of communication, such as magic slates, pen and pencil, and temporarily closing the opening over the trachea.

The primary postoperative goals are to maintain a patent airway, to prevent infection, and to allay the patient's apprehension, which increases the need for oxygen. Tracheotomy care is not particularly difficult, but meticulousness is a necessity. The copious secretions that result from infection further aggravate the patient. Some institutions employ the **clean technique** in care; others use the strict sterile technique, which is the one recommended by these authors. As techniques vary from institution to institution, the following discussion should be used only as a guide.

Tracheotomy care includes the use of the proper suctioning technique, cleansing around the outer tracheotomy tube and the inner cannula (if present), and the application of the dressing.

Suctioning

The purpose of suctioning is to withdraw secretions that the patient has difficulty expectorating. The equipment needed includes a sterile catheter, a Y-type tube, a vacuum suction pump, a single sterile glove, a sterile pan, and sterile water. The catheter is passed into the tracheotomy tube and into the trachea and, if deep suctioning is required, into the bronchi.

Procedure. After washing your hands, open the glove and the suction catheter packages. Put on the glove. To connect the catheter to the suction source, pull the cover off the suction catheter with the nonsterile hand, and grasp the catheter with the sterile gloved hand.

Leaving the suction off and the Y-tube open, insert the catheter down into the tracheotomy tube and into the trachea. (Closing off the Y-tube opening and suctioning during insertion may traumatize or tear the lining of the trachea.) After completely inserting the catheter, turn on the suctioning and slowly withdraw the catheter, rotating it in a circular motion as it is withdrawn. The circular motion enables more of the trachea to be suctioned. Do not use an up and down motion, because it may cause trauma. The entire procedure should not take more than *twenty seconds*. The time limit exists because of the dangers associated with hypoxia such as arrhythmias.

In order to reach both bronchi, ask the patient to turn his head to the left side to suction the right bronchus, and then to the right side to suction the left bronchus.

Administer oxygen to the patient between suctioning episodes to help maintain adequate ventilation.

One to three cubic centimeters of normal saline solution may be inserted into the trachea and suctioned immediately. This will help remove some of the more tenacious secretions. The frequency of suctioning will vary according to the need of the patient.

Cleaning the Tracheotomy Tube

Set up the tracheotomy cleaning set, which consists of containers for hydrogen peroxide and for sterile water, pipe cleaners, 2 x 2 dressings, and tracheotomy dressings. A sterile field is necessary. Hydrogen peroxide is recommended because it dissolves mucus secretions and bubbles by chemical action.

Fill the hydrogen peroxide container and the sterile water container. Having ready the suction catheter, glove both hands and suction the patient. Insure adequate oxygenation before beginning to clean the tubes.

If the set has one, remove the inner cannula. The nurse should *never* remove the outer cannula, unless it is specific hospital policy and the nurse has been properly instructed in the procedure. An extra tracheotomy tube, adaptor, and obturator should be kept at the bedside in case the tube is displaced. Place the inner cannula in the hydrogen peroxide and let it soak. If the patient has copious secretions, suction again. Then use a pipe cleaner to clean inside of the inner cannula. Rinse it with sterile normal saline or water and dry it with a pipe cleaner. Replace the inner cannula into the outer cannula. Clip the cannula in place and fasten the lock. Cleanse the outside of the tube and under the tube with a 2 x 2 dressing soaked in hydrogen peroxide.

Place the tracheotomy dressing slit upward and the telfa downward to keep the dressing from sticking to the wound. A double telfa dressing is ideal, since the secretions will slip off and not remain around the tube. Replace the ties. This should be done by two people so that the tracheotomy tube will not be coughed out while the ties are not secured.

Extended Nursing Care   Another aspect of nursing care for the patient with a tracheotomy tube is the humidification of the oxygen. Since the moisturizing part of the anatomy, the nose, is not functioning for this patient, intermittent positive pressure breathing (IPPB) may be recommended to loosen the secretions in the lungs to facilitate their removal. Chest physiotherapy and postural drainage may also be ordered. If not contraindicated, forcing fluids orally will help thin the secretions.

This patient must be supported emotionally and observed closely because of the fear of not being able to breathe. Means of communication need to be clearly established. Use of sedatives should be kept to a minimum because of the possibility of respiratory depression.

In preparation for a total closure, the physician will usually replace the tracheotomy tube with successively smaller sizes until the tube is finally removed. This process is called decannulization. Cultures may be taken to evaluate possible infection. The patient will need to relearn to breathe through the nose before the tube is completely removed.

BIBLIOGRAPHY

Brunner, L., et al.: Textbook of Medical-Surgical Nursing, ed. 3. J. B. Lippincott Company, Philadelphia, 1975.

Dison, N. G.: An Atlas of Nursing Techniques. The C. V. Mosby Company, St. Louis, 1971.

Fuerst, E. V., and Wolff, L.: Fundamentals of Nursing. J. B. Lippincott Company, Philadelphia, 1969.

Metheny, N. M., and Snively, W. D., Jr.: Nurses' Handbook of Fluid Balance, ed. 2. J. B. Lippincott Company, Philadelphia, 1974.

Sutton, A. L.: Bedside Nursing Techniques in Medicine and Surgery, ed. 2. W. B. Saunders Company, Philadelphia, 1969.

NOTES

NOTES

APPENDICES

1

Units of Measurement

METRIC SYSTEM

Weights

Scale	Table		Grams		Grains
Kilo	1 Kilogram	=	1000.0	=	15,432.35
Hecto	1 Hectogram	=	100.0	=	1,543.23
Deca	1 Decagram	=	10.0	=	154.323
Unit	1 Gram	=	1.0	=	15.432
Deci	1 Decigram	=	0.1	=	1.5432
Centi	1 Centigram	=	0.01	=	0.15432
Milli	1 Milligram	=	0.001	=	0.01543
Micro	1 Microgram	=	10^{-6}	=	15.432×10^{-6}
Nano	1 Nanogram	=	10^{-9}	=	15.432×10^{-9}
Pico	1 Picogram	=	10^{-12}	=	15.432×10^{-12}
Femto	1 Femtogram	=	10^{-15}	=	15.432×10^{-15}
Atto	1 Attogram	=	10^{-18}	=	15.432×10^{-18}

Arabic numbers are used with weights and measures, as 10 gm., or 3 ml., etc. Portions of weights and measures are usually expressed decimally. 10^{-1} indicates 1.0; 10^{-6}=0.000001; etc.

Tables of Data

Arabic numbers are used with weights and measures, as 10 gm., or 3 ml., etc. Portions of weights and measures are usually expressed decimally. For practical purposes, 1 cc. is equivalent to 1 ml. and 1 drop (gtt) of water is equivalent to a minim (m).

Units of Length

		Millimeters	Centimeters	Inches	Feet	Yards	Meters
1 mm.	=	1.0	0.1	0.03937	0.00328	0.0011	0.001
1 cm.	=	10.0	1.0	0.3937	0.03281	0.0109	0.01
1 in.	=	25.4	2.54	1.0	0.0833	0.0278	0.0254
1 ft.	=	304.8	30.48	12.0	1.0	0.333	0.3048
1 yd.	=	914.40	91.44	36.0	3.0	1.0	0.9144
1 m.	=	1000.0	100.0	39.37	3.2808	1.0936	1.0

1μ = 1 mu = 1 micron* = 0.001 millimeter. 1 mm. = 1000 μ.
1 km. = 1 kilometer = 1000 meters = 0.6215 mile.
1 mile = 5280 feet = 1.609 kilometers.
*Micron is also called micrometer. μm = 10^{-6}.

Appendix 1 is reprinted from Taber's Cyclopedic Medical Dictionary, ed. 13. Edited by Clayton L. Thomas. F. A. Davis Company, Philadelphia, 1977, Appendix pages 4 through 8.

Units of Volume (fluid or liquid)

		Milliliters	U.S. Fluid Drams	Cubic Inches	U.S. Fluid Ounces	U.S. Fluid Quarts	Liters
1 ml.	=	1.0	0.2705	0.061	0.03381	0.00106	0.001
1 fl. ℨ	=	3.697	1.0	0.226	0.125	0.00391	0.00369
1 cu. in.	=	16.3866	4.4329	1.0	0.5541	0.0173	0.01639
1 fl. ℥	=	29.573	8.0	1.8047	1.0	0.03125	0.02957
1 qt.	=	946.332	256.0	57.75	32.0	1.0	0.9463
1 L	=	1000.0	270.52	61.025	33.815	1.0567	1.0

1 gallon = 4 quarts = 8 pints = 3.785 liters.
1 pint = 473.16 ml.

Units of Weight

		Grains	Grams	Apothecaries Ounces	Avoirdupois Pounds	Kilograms
1 gr.	=	1.0	0.0648	0.00208	0.0001429	0.000065
1 gm.	=	15.432	1.0	0.03215	0.002205	0.001
1 ℥	=	480.0	31.1	1.0	0.06855	0.0311
1 lb.	=	7000.0	453.5924	14.583	1.0	0.45354
1 kg.	=	15432.358	1000.0	32.15	2.2046	1.0

1 γ = 1 gamma = 1 microgram = 0.001 milligram; 1000 γ = 1 mg.
1 mg. = 1 milligram = 0.001 gm.; 1000 mg. = 1 gm.
1 grain = 64.8 mg.; 1 mg. = 0.0154 grain.

Weights and Measures

Apothecaries' Weight

20 grains = 1 scruple
8 drams = 1 ounce

3 scruples = 1 dram
12 ounces = 1 pound

Avoirdupois Weight

27.343 grains = 1 dram
16 ounces = 1 pound
2000 pounds = 1 short ton
1 oz. troy = 480 grains
1 lb. troy = 5760 grains

16 drams = 1 ounce
100 pounds = 1 hundredweight
2240 pounds = 1 long ton
1 oz. avoirdupois = 437.5 grains
1 lb. avoirdupois = 7000 grains

Circular Measure

60 seconds = 1 minute
90 degrees = 1 quadrant

60 minutes = 1 degree
4 quadrants = 360 degrees = circle

Cubic Measure

1728 cubic inches = 1 cubic foot
2150.42 cubic inches = 1 standard bushel
1 cubic foot = about four-fifths of a bushel

27 cubic feet = 1 cubic yard
268.8 cubic inches = 1 dry (U.S.) gallon
128 cubic feet = 1 cord (wood)

Dry Measure

2 pints = 1 quart

8 quarts = 1 peck

4 pecks = 1 bushel

Liquid Measure

16 ounces = 1 pint
1000 milliliters = 1 liter
4 gills = 1 pint

2 pints = 1 quart
4 quarts = 1 gallon
31.5 gallons = 1 barrel (U.S.)

2 barrels = 1 hogshead (U.S.)
1 quart = 0.946 liters

Barrels and hogsheads vary in size. A U.S. gallon is equal to 0.8327 British gallon; therefore a British gallon is equal to 1.201 U.S. gallons.
1 liter is equal to 1.0567 quarts.

Linear Measure

1 inch = 2.54 centimeters
12 inches = 1 foot
1 statute mile = 5280 feet

40 rods = 1 furlong
3 feet = 1 yard
3 statute miles = 1 statute league

8 furlongs = 1 statute mile
5.5 yards = 1 rod

Troy Weight

24 grains = 1 pennyweight
20 pennyweights = 1 ounce
12 ounces = 1 pound
Used for weighing gold, silver, and jewels.

Household Measures* and Weights

Approximate Equivalents: 60 gtt. = 1 teaspoonful = 5 ml.
= 60 minims = 60 grains = 1 dram = ⅛ ounce

1 teaspoon = ⅛ fl. oz.; 1 dram	16 tablespoons (liquid) = 1 cup
3 teaspoons = 1 tablespoon	12 tablespoons (dry) = 1 cup
1 tablespoon = ½ fl. oz.; 4 drams	1 cup = 8 fl. oz.

1 tumbler or glass = 8 fl. oz.; ½ pint

*Household measures are not precise. For instance, household tsp. will hold from 3 to 5 ml. of liquid substances. Therefore, do not substitute household equivalents for medication prescribed by the physician.

CONVERSION RULES

To convert units of one system into the other, multiply the number of units in column I by the equivalent factor opposite that unit in column II.

Weight

I		II
1 milligram	=	0.015432 grain
1 gram	=	15.432 grains
1 gram	=	0.25720 apothecaries' dram
1 gram	=	0.03527 avoirdupois ounce
1 gram	=	0.03215 apothecaries' or troy ounce
1 kilogram	=	35.274 avoirdupois ounces
1 kilogram	=	32.151 apothecaries' or troy ounces
1 kilogram	=	2.2046 avoirdupois pounds
1 grain	=	64.7989 milligrams
1 grain	=	0.0648 gram
1 apothecaries' dram	=	3.8879 gram
1 avoirdupois ounce	=	28.3495 grams
1 apothecaries' or troy ounce	=	31.1035 grams
1 avoirdupois pound	=	453.5924 grams

Volume (air or gas)

I		II
1 cubic centimeter	=	0.06102 cubic inch
1 cubic meter	=	35.314 cubic feet
1 cubic meter	=	1.3079 cubic yard
1 cubic inch	=	16.3872 cubic centimeters
1 cubic foot	=	0.02832 cubic meter

Capacity (fluid or liquid)

I		II
1 milliliter	=	16.23 minims
1 milliliter	=	0.2705 fluid dram
1 milliliter	=	0.0338 fluid ounce
1 liter	=	33.8148 fluid ounces
1 liter	=	2.1134 pints
1 liter	=	1.0567 quart
1 liter	=	0.2642 gallon
1 fluid dram	=	3.697 milliliters
1 fluid ounce	=	29.573 milliliters
1 pint	=	473.166 milliliters
1 quart	=	946.332 milliliters
1 gallon	=	3.785 liters

To Convert Centigrade or Celsius Degrees to Fahrenheit Degrees
Multiply the number of Centigrade degrees by $9/5$ and add 32 to the result.
Example: 55° C. × $9/5$ = 99 + 32 = 131° F.
To Convert Fahrenheit Degrees to Centigrade Degrees
Subtract 32 from the number of Fahrenheit degrees and multiply the difference by $5/9$.
Example: 243° F. − 32 = 211 × $5/9$ = 117.2° C.

MISCELLANEOUS CONVERSION FACTORS

Pressure

to obtain	multiply	by
lb./sq. in.	atmospheres	14.696
lb./sq. in.	in. of water	0.03609
lb./sq. in.	ft. of water	0.4335
lb./sq. in.	in. of mercury	0.4912
lb./sq. in.	kg./sq. meter	0.00142
lb./sq. in.	kg./sq. cm.	14.22
lb./sq. in.	cm. of mercury	0.1934
lb./sq. ft.	atmospheres	2116.2
lb./sq. ft.	in. of water	5.1981
lb./sq. ft.	ft. of water	62.378
lb./sq. ft.	in of mercury	70.727
lb./sq. ft.	cm. of mercury	27.845
lb./sq. ft.	kg./sq. meter	0.20482
lb./cu. in.	gm./ml.	0.03613
lb./cu. ft.	lb./cu. in	1728.0
lb./cu. ft.	gm./ml.	62.428
lb./U.S. gal.	gm./ml.	8.345
in. of water	in. of mercury	13.60
in. of water	cm. of mercury	5.3524
ft. of water	atmospheres	33.93
ft. of water	lb./sq. in.	2.311
ft. of water	kg./sq. meter	0.00328
ft. of water	in. of mercury	1.133
ft. of water	cm. of mercury	0.4460
atmospheres	ft. of water	0.02947
atmospheres	in. of mercury	0.03342
atmospheres	kg./sq. cm.	0.9678
bars	atmospheres	1.0133
in. of mercury	atmospheres	29.921
in. of mercury	lb./sq. in.	2.036
mm. of mercury	atmospheres	760.0
gm./ml.	lb./cu. in.	27.68
gm./sq. cm.	lb./sq. in.	70.31
gm./sq. cm.	kg./sq. meter	0.1
kg./sq. meter	in. of water	25.38
kg./sq. meter	in. of mercury	345.32
kg./sq. meter	cm. of mercury	135.95
kg./sq. meter	atmospheres	10332.0
kg./sq. cm.	atmospheres	1.0332

Flow Rate

To obtain	multiply	by
cu. ft./hr.	cc./min.	0.00212
cu. ft./hr.	L./min.	2.12
L./min.	cu. ft./hr.	0.472

Parts Per Million

Conversion of parts per million (ppm) to percent: 1 ppm = 0.0001%, 10 ppm = 0.001%, 100 ppm = 0.01%, 1000 ppm = 0.1%, 10,000 ppm = 1%, etc.

2

Laboratory Values

Following is a list of normal laboratory values used throughout this text. *Laboratory values may differ slightly among the various institutions.*

HEMATOLOGY

Blood count (red)	F 3.8-5.8 million/cu mm
	M 4.4-6.4 million/cu mm
Blood count (white)	5,000-10,000/cu mm
HCT	F 37-47% M 40-54%
Hgb	F 11-15 gm % M 12-17 gm %

URINE CHEMISTRY

Addis count, RBCs	Less than one half million
WBCs	Less than one million
Casts	Less than 5,000 (hyaline)
Calcium	50-300 mg per 24 hours
Catecholamines	Up to 100 mEq per 24 hours
Chlorides	170-250 mEq per 24 hours
Creatinine clearance	100-130 cc/min
LDH (lactic dehydrogenase) ..	0-8,000 units
17-OH corticosteroids	5.5-12 mg/24 hours (adult)
	3mg/24 hours (up to 10 years)
17-ketosteroids	5-15 mg/24 hours (female)
	7-20 mg/24 hours (male)
	21 mg/24 hours (children under 6)
	3mg/24 hours (6–10 years)
Potassium	27-123 mEq/24 hours
Sodium	43-217 mEq/24 hours
Specific gravity	1.015-1.025
Sugar (quan.)	negative
Urea clearance	Standard 40-68 cc/min
Urea nitrogen	2.7-9.9 gms/24 hours
Uric acid	600 mg/L
Urine osmolality	270-900 mOsm/kg; mean 550 mOsm/kg

BLOOD CHEMISTRY

Blood urea nitrogen (BUN) ...	10-20 mg%
Calcium	8.5-10.5 mg%
Chloride	95-105 mEq/L
CO_2	24-32 mEq/L (adults)
	18-27 mEq/L (children)
Creatinine	0.5-1.5 mg/100 ml
Creatinine clearance	100-130 cc/min
Electrolytes: sodium (Na)	135-145 mEq/L
potassium (K) ...	3.5-5.0 mEq/L
chloride (Cl)	95-105 mEq/L
CO_2	24-32 mEq/L
Glucose (fasting)	65-110 mg%
Lactic dehydrogenase (LDH) ..	100-225 Technicon units
Osmolality	275-300 mOsm/kg
Phosphorous	2.5-4.5 mg
Potassium	3.5-5.0 mEq/L
Protein	6.8 gm%
Sodium	135-145 mEq/L
Urea clearance	Standard 40-68 cc/min
	Maximal 64-99 cc/min
Uric acid	2.5-8.0 mg%
Total protein	Under 0.15 gms/24 hours

BLOOD GASES

	Mean	Range
pH	V:7.37	(7.32-7.42)
	A:7.40	(7.35-7.45)
pCO_2	V:46	(42-55) mmHg
	A:40	(34-46)mmHg
H_2CO_3	V:1.38	(1.26-1.65) mm/L
	A:1.20	(1.02-1.38)mm/L
HCO_3	V:26	(24-28) mEq/L
	A:24	(22-26) mEq/L
pO_2	V:40	(Varies with pH) mmHg
	A:90	
O_2 Sat	V:62	(55-71) %
	A:98	(over 90) %

3

Fluid and Electrolyte
Intake and Output Record

Date _____

INTAKE									OUTPUT					
Time	IV NO.	Intravenous	Amt. in bottle	Amt. taken	Time	Oral/Gastric	Amt.	Irrig.	Time	Urine	Emesis	Suction	Diaphoresis
					7:00AM	milk	230						
8:00 AM	#1	D5/½ NS	1000	1000					9:00 AM	400			
					12:30	milk	100		1:30 PM	150			
7-3 Totals				1000			330			550			
4:00 PM	#2	D5/½ NS + 40 mEq KCL	1000	800					5:00 PM	200			
									8:00 PM	400			
3-11 Totals				800			0			600			
12:00 MN	#3	D5/½ NS + 20 mEq KCL	1000	1000					2:00 AM	300			
									6:00 AM	300			
11-7 Totals				1000			0			600			
24 Hour Totals				2800			330			1750			

4

Case Study Discussions

1. ECF excess: orthopnea, shortness of breath, and edema
2. a. ECF excess: In congestive heart failure, decreased cardiac output causes a decreased renal blood flow with resulting sodium and water retention.
   b. Potassium deficit: Diuretic therapy increases loss of potassium which may result in a potassium deficit. KCl was ordered in anticipation of a potassium deficit (See Chapter 5).
3. HCT 31% is decreased. The hematocrit measures per cent of volume and thus will be decreased with an increased amount of extracellular fluid. BUN is slightly elevated. This indicates prerenal **azotemia** from a poor glomerular filtration rate due to the heart problem. Cl 90.8 is decreased. The chloride excretion is increased, as the diuretics have increased urine output. K 3.1 is decreased. This is due to diuresis and poor intake of nutrients.
4. Because the HCT measures per cent of volume, with the four pound loss of fluid, the hematocrit rose porportionately.

1. a. ECF deficit: vomiting, weight loss, anorexia, diarrhea, weakness, decreased blood pressure
   b. Potassium deficit: vomiting, anorexia, diarrhea, weakness (see Chapter 5)
2. Vomitus: 50-100 mEq/L of sodium and chloride
   Diarrhea: 30-50 mEq/L of sodium and chloride
3. Serum sodium 121 is decreased and indicates a water excess (see Chapter 3).
   Chloride 82 is decreased and usually increases or decreases in proportion to the serum sodium.
   CO_2 9 is decreased and indicates an acidosis (see Chapter 10). The patient is retaining hydrogen ions (H_+) because he has not urinated for 4 days. Retention of these fixed acids causes renal acidosis.
   BUN 139 is elevated and indicates a renal failure. This patient is retaining the nitrogenous waste products and has become azotemic. The ECF deficit is so severe that the kidneys are not getting sufficient

intravascular supply to function properly, thus resulting in oliguria. Hematocrit 57% is increased. Hematocrit is measured in per cent of volume and thus will be increased with a decreased amount of ECF.
4. No
5. a. Intake-Output (*hourly* output) Record
   b. BP at least every two hours (postural, if condition permits); vital signs
   c. NPO pending physician orders. Fluid restriction is the treatment for the intracellular excess which has been noted by the serum sodium report of 121.
6. Dextrose 5% in normal saline. This fluid will go into the extracellular fluid compartment and correct the saline depletion. The physician will correct only one-half of the deficit in the first 24 hours and the other half over several days.

Case Study 3.1

1. ECF deficit: weakness, vomiting, weight loss
   ICF excess: headache
   Potassium deficit: weakness, vomiting (see Chapter 5).
   Metabolic alkalosis; vomiting (see Chapter 10)
2. Decreased RBC, Hgb, and HCT; cause unknown; possible hemorrhage, poor nutrition. Elevated BUN indicates azotemia.
3. a) Notify physician; b) initiate intake-output record; c) measure and record daily weight and BP.
4. BUN 80: elevated and rising. Lack of urination has resulted in retention of waste products.
   Serum sodium 121: decreased; reveals an increase in total body water. The solute is diluted in an excessive amount of water.
   Chloride 85: low; related to serum sodium.
   CO_2 14: decreased; indicates metabolic acidosis or decreased bicarbonate. Metabolic acidosis is caused by abnormal metabolism due to impaired excretion of fixed acids. This patient has uremic acidosis.
5. Yes. Serious problems can develop from rapid water and electrolyte loss. Postural blood pressure should be taken and patient observed for signs of hypovolemia (ECF deficit). The previous serum sodium reading was 121, indicating a water excess. It is now 142, indicating loss of total body water.
6. BUN is being removed with kidney excretion. The kidneys are able to function after relief of obstruction. Fixed acids are excreted and acidosis corrected.

Case Study 3.2

1. a) Intracellular fluid deficit; b) potassium deficit.
2. Intracellular fluid deficit:
   weakness
   restlessness
   flushed skin
   dulled sensorium
   elevated temperature
   Potassium deficit:
   malnourished
   weakness
3. Na: elevated
   Cl: elevated

K: decreased

BUN: elevated

4. (Yes or no according to the correctness of your answer.) The report supports a diagnosis of intracellular fluid and potassium deficits.
5. a) Notify the physician; b) force fluids; c) record intake and output.
6. There is insufficient blood volume to excrete the urea normally.

Case Study 4

1. The drop in the systolic pressure is indicative of an ECF deficit. The patient's strict adherence to the low sodium diet plus the over-zealous use of diuretics had induced a hypovolemic state. ADH output will be increased.
2. Na 114 indicates a water excess. This low serum sodium level is *frequently* but *erroneously* related to sodium need. The saline deficit has caused an ADH increase with the subsequent retention of water. These two problems, saline deficit and water excess, need to be treated *separately*.

   Cl 72 indicates a decrease and is in proportion to the serum sodium.

   K 2.4 indicates a severe decrease. Thiazide diuretics promote potassium excretion. A potassium level this low needs immediate correction and should be brought up to at least 3.0 within 18 to 24 hours.

   CO_2 18 indicates acidosis. The hypovolemic state has caused the oliguria leading to retention of metabolic waste products, such as urea, inorganic acids, and phosphoric and sulfuric acids. Urea is the end product of protein metabolism.

   BUN 60 indicates a renal problem with some azotemia.

Case Study 5.1

1. As urine output decreases, the body retains the metabolic waste products, such as urea; thus the BUN level rises. The body maintains potassium balance by excreting the excess. As urine excretion decreases, the serum potassium level rises.
2. Yes. This patient suffered severe tissue destruction due to her injuries. Since 98 per cent of the body's potassium is intracellular, the tissue trauma would precipitate the movement of potassium into the extra-cellular compartment.
3. No. The nurse did not recognize the emergency situation.
4. The Na lactate, an alkaline solution, would be antagonistic and reverse the effect on the heart caused by the elevated potassium. The glucose and insulin would drive the potassium back into the cells (intracellular compartment) where it is non-toxic. It must be remembered that this is a temporary emergency procedure until the excess potassium is removed from the body by other means, such as peritoneal or hemodialysis.
5. Tented T waves, or elevated T waves are most common. Other variations include: widened QRS, absent P waves.

Case Study 5.2

1. Potassium and chloride.
2. The physician should be notified immediately because a patient with a potassium depletion this severe could develop cardiac arrhythmias or flaccid paralysis with paralysis of the respiratory muscles and resulting death.
3. Blood pressure and pulse should be taken every 3 to 4 hours with the

nurse being alert to changes such as hypotension and irregularities in the pulse rate.
4. The usual amount of KCl is 40 mEq/L. The usual rate of flow is not over 20 mEq/L of KCl per hour.
5. Depressed T waves, possibly U waves, prolonged Q-T segment, and depressed S-T segments.

Case Study 10.1

1. Water tends to be retained to maintain extracellular fluid and blood volume; this results in low serum sodium and serum chloride readings.
2. Hyperglycemia increases urinary output by acting as an osmotic diuretic. The increased sugar in the serum is a hypertonic solution and pulls the water to it.
3. Blood sugar 454: elevated and requiring immediate and continuing attention.
   CO_2 11: indicates metabolic acidosis.
   Na 130: decreased; indicates water excess.
   Cl 93: decreased and in proportion to Na.
   K 7.6: increased and requiring emergency treatment. Potassium rises in acidosis because as the excess hydrogen ions move into the cell, potassium moves out into the serum.
   pH 7.27: indicates an acidosis, in this case metabolic, requiring emergency attention.
   pCO_2 24: indicates respiratory compensation for metabolic acidosis.
   HCO_3 13.5: indicates deficit of bicarbonate and metabolic acidosis.
   pO_2 91: normal.
4. The low CO_2 indicates metabolic acidosis from ketone acids. Ketone acids are end products of fat metabolism. Fats metabolize because glucose cannot be metabolized without sufficient insulin. Acetone is a ketone. This patient has ketoacidosis.
5. Administration of insulin would stop the production of ketone bodies. Sodium bicarbonate helps restore base balance.

Case Study 10.2

1. Saline (ECF) deficit: vomiting, gastric suction, paralytic ileus (which has a third space effect in that fluid is isolated in the body and not physiologically available).
   Alkalosis: elevated CO_2; history of gastrointestinal loss.
   Potassium deficit: laxative abuse, diarrhea, vomiting, and gastric suction.
   Chloride deficit: vomiting, gastric suction.
2. Sodium decreased: indicates water (ICF) excess. Water is retained in an attempt to maintain the extracellular fluid and therefore the intracellular fluid volume.
   Potassium decreased: potassium decreases in alkalosis (note CO_2 of 44).
   Chloride decreased: out of proportion to the serum sodium deficit, indicating hypochloremic metabolic alkalosis.
   Carbon dioxide elevated: indicates excess bicarbonate (metabolic alkalosis).
3. 30 cc of normal saline solution. Levin tube irrigation with water would further deplete electrolytes. Water, which is hypotonic, draws sodium chloride and potassium from the extracellular compartment into the stomach or bowel while establishing equilibrium of the solutes, so that

isotonicity is achieved. Patients on gastrointestinal suction should not be allowed water and ice because these liquids promote excessive intestinal secretion and loss of electrolytes. When the physician orders sips of water and ice chips, they should be very carefully regulated and accurately measured. All gastrointestinal losses should also be carefully measured.

4. This patient has metabolic alkalosis. Sustained metabolic alkalosis can only occur in the presence of an increased renal threshold for bicarbonate, permitting a high level of bicarbonate to be maintained. Clinically, this situation occurs when chloride depletion is out of proportion to sodium depletion or when severe potassium depletion occurs. Such a circumstance may result from (a) loss of hydrochloric acid by vomiting or gastric suction or (b) loss of potassium chloride.

Case Study 11.1

1. a. Make a nursing assessment. The nurse would learn that this patient had a history of chronic obstructive pulmonary disease (COPD). He had been ill at home for four weeks with an upper respiratory infection exhibiting a cough, dyspnea, and low grade fever. The nurse observed that he was having difficulty with aeration, appeared exhausted and somnolent.
   b. Report observations to physician.
   c. Alert the nursing staff that this patient had three of the major precipitating factors that can lead to acute respiratory failure: (1) COPD; (2) acute infection; (3) order for sedation.
2. Yes. This patient is very susceptible to a CO_2 narcosis. Too much O_2 will remove the stimulus of oxygen deficiency which causes the medulla to maintain normal breathing. It is preferable to maintain adequate oxygenation with a low flow of O_2 (1 to 2 L/min).
3. Change the patient's position, encourage frequent coughing and deep breathing, maintain proper hydration, and teach proper breathing techniques.
4. a. Aminophyllin is a smooth muscle relaxant indicated in this case for its action on the bronchial muscle and coronary arteries. Since it can cause convulsions it should *never* be given faster than one cc per minute.
   b. Na 143: normal
      K 5.3: normal
      Cl 104: normal
      CO_2 44: elevated (usually found in COPD compensation)
      BUN 16: normal
      pH 7.27: decreased indicating an acidosis (life-threatening and requiring immediate and continuous attention)
      pCO_2 72: elevated indicating respiratory acidosis (life-threatening)
      pO_2 108: elevated (previous O_2 order of 5 L was decreased to 1 L/min)
5. Sedatives are one of the most common causes of death in acute respiratory failure because they depress respiration and thus increase pCO_2 further.
6. The potassium is elevated but is still within the normal range because this patient's potassium was severely decreased before the acidosis developed. The nurse should be very alert to the possibility of the potassium decreasing as the acidosis is corrected. A critically low level requires immediate correction.
7. This patient was so sensitive to oxygen that he could not even tolerate

the 40 per cent oxygen used during the IPPB treatment. He satisfactorily responded to IPPB treatment with compressed air. With proper treatment and nursing care, this patient was dismissed in four weeks. Increased ventilation corrected the acidosis. Treatment also included intravenous fluids, antibiotics, steroids, IPPB treatments followed by postural drainage and percussion, and breathing exercises. The decreased potassium was corrected by oral administration and diet.

Case Study 11.2

1. pH 7.58: elevated; indicates alkalosis.
   pCO_2 22: decreased; indicates respiratory alkalosis.
   pO_2 77: slightly decreased and non-alarming
   BUN 64, creatinine 2.5: both are elevated and show decreased renal function with some azotemia.
2. Hyperventilation is rapid breathing causing excessive amounts of carbon dioxide to be "blown off." There is increased alveolar ventilation in relation to the metabolic rate.
3. No. Hypoxia is a condition where there is a low oxygen content in the body. Ventilation is the process of moving gases into and out of the alveoli. The level of pCO_2 is a measure of this function.
4. Sedation and/or reassurance.
5. Patients on mechanical ventilators often develop iatrogenic respiratory alkalosis. It is imperative that an inhalation therapist remain in constant attendance and that blood gases tests are taken frequently until the machine becomes satisfactorily regulated to the patient. The heart does not tolerate alkalosis well.

Case Study 14

1. A mismatched blood transfusion causes hemolysis and the obstruction of the kidney vessels and/or tubules from agglutination of the red blood cells.
2. The kidneys are not able to reabsorb sodium.
3. The cardiac monitor was required because of the elevated potassium level. It is extremely important to watch for EKG changes as these may be the only warning of cardiac arrest. The EKG changes to watch for are: elevated, tented T waves, widened QRS, prolonged P-R waves, ST segment depression, absent P wave, atrial arrest, and sine wave.
4. Her fluid intake would be calculated from the estimated insensible loss (approximately 800 cc), minus 400 cc from catabolism, which would total approximately 400 cc/24 hours. When the patient developed diaphoresis, fluids were increased accordingly. This calculation was made from the nurse's records.

   The patient was given a high fat, high carbohydrate diet. The carbohydrates were given for their protein sparing effect.

   Calories were provided with IV administration of a 20 per cent glucose solution.
5. Fresh packed cells were used because of their lower potassium content. Older blood has a higher potassium content as a result of cellular breakdown.

Case Study 15

1. Chronic renal disease.
2. Hemoglobin and hematocrit readings are decreased. Anemia is a complication of chronic renal disease. Toxic products prevent the bone

marrow from releasing red blood cells or producing blood adequately. Blood has also been lost due to the hematemesis. Patients with these problems develop complications with platelets and blood vessels (usually intestinal). The reason for the defect is unknown. BUN and creatinine are elevated, indicating that the acidosis is renal. Sodium and chloride are slightly elevated. CO_2 is decreased, indicating metabolic acidosis.

The urine RBC reading of 1-10 is significant of chronic renal disease. The entire urinalysis is abnormal. The casts are formed from protein and can indicate kidney pathology. The albumin reading indicates that the glomeruli, normally impermeable to protein, are leaking protein.

3. Vital signs qid
   Accurate intake-output record
   Accurate daily weight
4. Patients with chronic renal disease usually maintain a stable potassium balance until the terminal stage. The main problem is the inability to excrete urea and creatinine, not potassium.
5. The fluid intake will be determined by the physician after he computes the sensible and insensible losses. An accurate intake-output record is essential for this calculation.
6. Patients with chronic renal disease are usually placed on a low protein, high caloric diet. The exact diet is determined on an individual basis. Approximately 80 per cent of these patients will also be on a sodium restricted diet because they are "salt-retainers." It is important that the 20 per cent who are "salt-losers" be recognized so they are not treated as "salt-retainers." Since this patient's disease was quite advanced and she had no evidence of edema, she was probably a mild "salt-loser."

   There is a definite correlation between life span and adherence to the diet.

Case Study 18

1. Extracellular fluid deficit; chloride depletion (metabolic alkalosis); potassium depletion.
2. 50 to 100 mEq/L sodium, 100 mEq/L chloride, 5 to 10 mEq/L potassium.
3. Notify the physician of the patient's poor response. Improvement can be anticipated if the treatment is adequate.
4. The patient will lose electrolytes and large amounts of fluid. Each episode of diaphoresis requiring a linen change represents about 1000 cc of fluid lost. Diaphoresis may be a sign of shock. A decrease in blood pressure activates receptor sites which stimulate the sympathetic nervous system to release catecholamines (epinephrine and norepinephrine). Catecholamines stimulate the sweat glands.
5. Mannitol expands plasma volume and is an osmotic diuretic. It is desired that the increased blood flow will perfuse the kidneys and consequently improve kidney function. The patient's response to Mannitol will indicate whether the patient has prerenal or intrarenal (parenchymal) failure. If an adequate urinary output develops (over 300 cc/3 hours), the patient has prerenal failure. Little or minimal response to Mannitol indicates intrarenal failure.
6. Na 122: decreased, indicating water excess. Patient is receiving intravenous fluids but not voiding adequately due to the oliguria.

Cl 86: decreased from loss in gastric suction and also in proportion to the serum sodium.

CO_2 9 and pH 7.20: decreased, indicating renal metabolic acidosis.

BUN 188 and creatinine 10: Patient is unable to excrete metabolic waste products due to oliguric condition.

5

Answers to Quizzes

1. (c) ECF excess   2. (b) ECF decreased   3. No   4. True   5. True

1. (a) Decreased   2. (c) None   3. True   4. (b) Urine output less than 20 cc/hr, 160 cc/8 hrs, 480 cc/24 hrs.   5. True   6. True

1. Na^+ 50-100 mEq/L; Cl^- 100 mEq/L; K^+ 5-10 mEq/L.   2. False   3. True
4. Intracellular fluid excess.

1. Water: decreased. Saline: normal. Potassium: decreased. BUN: increased.   2. Serum sodium test.   3. Water replacement—either orally or intravenously.   4. True   5. True

1. (a) take daily weight; (c) notify physician; (d) restrict fluids; (e) measure hourly urine output; (f) record intake and output; (g) observe and record vital signs q 4 hours (including postural blood pressure).   2. water excess   3. Since water passes freely across cell membranes into the cells, excessive water in the brain cells causes them to swell.   4. (a) False   (b) True   (c) True   (d) True   (e) True

1. BUN — increased. Serum K — increased.   2. By excreting the excess potassium through the urine.   3. 6 mEq/L   4. True   5. (1) Renal failure; (2) acidosis; (3) intravenous fluid with potassium administered too rapidly.

1. Saline: normal or decreased (no HCT level to verify; history supports decrease). Water: normal. Potassium: decreased.   2. True   3. (b) respiratory paralysis progressing to arrhythmias.   4. No. Potassium should never be given as a direct undiluted injection.   5. 3.0 mEq/L.

Quiz 10.1

1. True 2. True 3. True 4. True 5. True 6. True 7. True
8. False

Quiz 10.2

1. ECF (saline): decreased. Na (water): increased. K: decreased. Cl: decreased. CO_2:increased. 2. a. (1) normal saline. b. (2) minimal amounts of water and ice chips because liquids promote excessive intestinal secretion and loss of electrolytes. 3. (b) excess of bicarbonate. 4. (d) pH 7.50 pCO_2 45 pO_2 86 HCO_3 38

Quiz 11.1

1. False 2. True 3. True 4. True 5. False 6. True 7. False 8. (a) airway obstruction. 9. (b) airway obstruction. 10. (b) diffusion defect. 11. (b) diffusion defect. 12. (c) perfusion problem.

Quiz 11.2

1. alkalosis 2. (a) False (b) True (c) True (d) True 3. Respiratory acidosis — (e) pH 7.15, pCO_2 60, pO_2 40, HCO_3 39; Metabolic acidosis — (b) pH 7.15, pCO_2 24, pO_2 88, HCO_3 8; Respiratory alkalosis — (d) pH 7.52, pCO_2 24, pO_2 88, HCO_3 22; Metabolic alkalosis — (a) pH 7.52, pCO_2 45, pO_2 88, HCO_3 36.

Quiz 14

1. True 2. True 3. False 4. False 5. False 6. True 7. False
8. False 9. True 10. True

Quiz 15

1. Vomiting blood. 2. Renal metabolic. 3. (a) True (b) True (c) True (d) True (e) True (f) True 4. The serum creatinine and 24-hour creatinine clearance test. 5. False 6. (b) low protein, high caloric diet.

Quiz 18

1. True 2. False 3. True 4. False 5. True 6. False 7. True 8. True
9. True 10. False

Glossary

acidosis. A disturbance of the acid-base balance of the body resulting in an acid condition in the serum; a pH below 7.35.

ADH. Abbr. for antidiuretic hormone.

aldosterone. A hormone produced by the adrenal cortex which regulates the volume of blood and extracellular water through the reabsorption of sodium by the kidneys.

alkalosis. Increase in body alkalinity resulting in a base excess in the serum; a pH above 7.45.

alveoli. Microscopic air cells in the lungs.

anaerobic. Having the ability to live without air.

anasarca. Generalized massive edema.

anion. A negatively charged ion. Examples are: Cl^-, HCO_3^-, HPO_4^-, lactate.

anorexia. Loss of appetite.

anoxia. Absence of oxygen in the body tissues.

antidiuretic hormone. A hormone produced by the hypothalamus and secreted by the pituitary gland that suppresses the secretion of urine and results in the retention of water. Abbr.: ADH.

anuria. Urine output less than 10 cc/24 hours.

apnea. Cessation of respiration in the resting expiratory position.

arrhythmia. Abnormal rhythm of the heart.

ascites. Serous fluid in the peritoneal cavity.

asterixis. A motor disturbance marked by inability to maintain an assumed posture as a result of intermittency of the sustained contraction of groups of muscles; flapping tremors of the extremities.

asthenia. Lack or loss of strength.

azotemia. Presence of increased nitrogenous waste products in the blood (azo = nitrogen; emia = blood).

bicarbonate. A salt resulting from the incomplete neutralization of carbonic acid or from the passing of an excess of carbon dioxide into a solution of a base; HCO_3^-. Syn.: base.

Biot's respiration. Originally described in patients with meningitis; refers to sequences of uniformly deep gasps alternating with apnea.

buffer. A chemical substance that reacts to variations in the serum alkalinity/acidity in such a way that changes in the pH level are minimized; it also acts as a transport system that moves excess H ions to the lung.

buffer base. Any substance that will neutralize an acid substance; correlates with alkali.

cachectic. Malnourished.

cardiac insufficiency. Inadequate cardiac output due to failure of the heart to function properly; pump failure.

cardiogenic. Having origin in the heart.

catabolism. The breaking down of living cells or nutrients into simpler substances, most of which are excreted.

catecholamines. The hormones epinephrine and norepinephrine produced by the sympathetic nervous system.

cation. A positively charged ion. Examples are: Na^+, K^+, Ca^{++}, Mg^{++}.

Cheyne-Stokes respirations. Cycles of gradually increasing tidal volume followed by gradually decreasing tidal volume, followed by apnea.

chloride. A chemical compound that is one of the major anions of the extracellular fluid; it functions to maintain the osmotic pressure of the blood.

cirrhosis. An interstitial inflammation with hardening, granulation, and contraction of the tissues of the liver.

clean technique. A procedure that renders a surface free, as nearly as possible, from pathogenic micro-organisms.

colloid. Gelatinous substance; opposite of crystalloid; a particle invisible to the naked eye which instead of dissolving is held in a state of suspension.

compensation. The counterbalancing of any defect of structure or function.

compensation, metabolic. A body function in which lungs balance pH partially or completely. In metabolic acidosis, the lungs hyperventilate to "blow off" acid (pCO_2); in metabolic alkalosis, the lungs hypoventilate to retain acid.

compensation, respiratory. A body function in which kidneys balance the pH partially or completely. In respiratory acidosis, the kidneys retain bicarbonate (HCO_3^-) and excrete excess hydrogen ions; in respiratory alkalosis the kidneys retain the excess hydrogen ions.

COP. Abbr. for colloid osmotic pressure; that component of the osmotic pressure supplied by large protein molecules, especially albumin.

COPD. Abbr. for chronic obstructive pulmonary disease.

cor pulmonale. Heart disease due to lung disease.

crenation. The reduction of a red blood cell due to mixture with a hypertonic solution.

CRF. Abbr. for corticotrophic releasing factor.

crystalloid. Clear like a crystal; opposite of colloid; a substance capable of crystallization which in solution can be diffused through animal membranes and is readily soluble, e.g., salt, sugar.

cubital fossa. The furrow in the elbow area.

diaphoresis. Profuse sweating, causing loss of fluid and electrolytes.

diffusion. Movement of solutes or gases from an area of higher concentration to an area of lower concentration; a passive transport system.

diuretic. Increasing or an agent which increases the excretion of urine.

dysphagia. Difficulty in swallowing.

dyspnea. Labored or difficult breathing.

ecchymosis. Blood under the skin; a bruise.

ECF. Abbr. for extracellular fluid.

edema. A condition in which the interstitial (tissue) spaces contain an excessive amount of extracellular fluid.

edema, dependent. The collection of extracellular fluid in interstitial spaces secondary to gravitational flow.

edema, pitting. The collection of extracellular fluid in tissue spaces without gravity flow. Finger impressions remain when applied pressure is released.

electrolyte. A substance capable of dissociating into ions and which in solution will conduct an electric current.

erythropoietin. A hormone produced by the kidney which stimulates red blood cell production in the bone marrow.

extracellular. Any area inside the body but outside the cell; interstitial and intravascular areas.

extracellular fluid. A chemical solution, primarily saline, which occupies the areas outside the cells. Abbr.: ECF.

Fe. Chemical symbol for iron.

febrile. Feverish; having a high body temperature.

fibrillation. Tremor or rapid action of the heart without effective cardiac output.

filtration. A passive transport system.

gavage. A feeding administered into the stomach via a nasogastric or orogastric tube.

GFR. Abbr. for glomerular filtration rate.

glucocorticoids. Hormones of the steroid class secreted by the adrenal cortex.

HCT. Abbr. for hematocrit.

hematemesis. Vomiting of blood.

hematocrit. A laboratory test evaluating the relationship between erythrocyte plasma and content of blood. Abbr.: HCT.

hematogenic. Pertaining to the formation of blood.

hemoconcentration. An increase in the number of red blood cells resulting from a decrease in the volume of plasma.

hemolysis. The enlargement of a red blood cell to a swollen globular state due to mixture with a hypotonic saline solution or distilled water.

hemoptysis. Blood-tinged sputum arising from hemorrhage of larynx, trachea, bronchi, or lungs.

Henderson-Hasselbach Equation. $pH = 6.1 + \underset{10}{LOG} \frac{HCO_3^-}{H_2CO_3}$

Hgb. Abbr. for hemoglobin.

homeostasis. The integrated balance of all body systems.

HPF. Abbr. for high-powered field (microscopic).

hydrogen ions. See: ions, hydrogen.

hydrostatic pressure. Pressure exerted on liquids and pressure of liquids in equilibrium.

hypercalcemia. Excessive calcium in the blood.

hypercapnia. Excessive carbon dioxide in the blood.

hyperchloremia. Excessive chloride in the blood.

hyperkalemia. Excessive potassium in the blood.

hypernatremia. Excessive sodium in the blood.

hyperpnea. Increased breathing; usually refers to increased tidal volume with or without increased frequency.

hyperreflexia. Increased action of the reflexes.

hypertonic. A solution that has a higher osmotic pressure than the one to which it is compared.

hypertonicity. (1) Excess muscular tonus; (2) a solution with greater osmotic pressure or concentration of solutes than blood.

hyperventilation. Respirations which are rapid and increased both in depth and rate causing a deficit of pCO_2^-. Syn.: hyperpnea.

hypervolemia. Abnormal increase in the volume of circulating fluid in the body.

hypocalcemia. Decreased calcium in the blood.

hypochloremia. Decreased chloride in the blood.

hypokalemia. Decreased potassium in the blood.

hyponatremia. Decreased sodium in the blood.

hypoproteinemia. Decrease in the normal quantity of protein (usually albumin and globulin) in the blood.

hyporeflexia. Diminished function of the reflexes.

hypothalmic. Pertaining to the hypothalmus.

hypotonic. A solution with a lower osmotic pressure than the one to which it is compared.

hypoventilation. Decreased alveolar ventilation in relation to metabolic rate.

hypovolemia. Diminished circulating blood volume.

hypoxemia. Inadequate oxygenation of the blood.

ICF. Abbr. for intracellular fluid.

iatrogenic. Resulting from treatment by the physician.

infarction. Cessation of the blood supply with resultant death to the tissue of an organ; usually results from vascular occlusion or stenosis.

inspiratory stridor. A harsh, high-pitched sound usually due to obstruction in the air passages.

insensible loss. Loss of body fluids which occur without the individual's awareness.

integumentary. Related to integument. Syn.: skin.

interstitial. The area between and around the cells.

interstitial fluid. Extracellular fluid composed of water and electrolytes which circulates between and around the cells.

intracellular. Area within the cell.

intracellular fluid. A solution of water and electrolytes which circulates within the cell. Abbr.: ICF.

intravascular. Within the blood vessels.

ion. An electrically charged particle.

ion, hydrogen. An electrically charged hydrogen molecule

ionize. The process by which an electrically charged chemical moves from one chemical compound to another.

IPPB. Abbr. for intermittent positive pressure breathing.

ischemia. Localized tissue anemia due to obstruction of the inflow of arterial blood.

isosthenuria. "Poor urine"; little variation in the urinary specific gravity of a person with nephritis.

isotonic. A solution having the same osmotic pressure as the one to which it is compared.

kg, 75. The weight of an average-sized man (165 pounds). See kilogram.

kilogram. A weight measurement equal to 2.2 pounds. Abbr.: kg.

Krebs' cycle. Citric acid cycle.

KVO. Abbr. for keep vein open.

lactic acid. A colorless syrupy liquid ($C_3H_6O_3$) formed in muscles during activity by the breakdown of glycogen (glycolysis) during the anaerobic cycle.

lactic dehydrogenase. An enzyme released from injury in selected organs, especially the heart and liver. Abbr.: LDH.

laryngectomy. Removal of the larynx.

lavage. Washing out of the stomach via intubation.

LDH. Abbr. for lactic dehydrogenase.

mOsm. Abbr. for milliosmol. A measure of solute concentration expressed at 1/1000th of the molar (or molal) concentration of an equivalent "perfect solute."

melena. Blood in the feces.

milliequivalent. A measurement of solutes in terms of combining power; the weight of a substance contained in one milliliter of a normal saline solution. Abbr.: mEq.

mineralcorticoid. A hormone of the steroid group, produced by the adrenal cortex.

molecule. The smallest division of a chemical compound possible without altering its original characteristics.

morbidity. Disease state.

mortality. Death rate.

narcosis. A reversible condition characterized by stupor or insensibility.

nephron. The functional unit of the kidney.

nephrosis. Condition in which there are degenerative changes in the kidneys without the occurrence of inflammation.

neurogenic. Originating from nervous tissue.

nonelectrolyte. Substances such as sugar or urea which in solution do not dissociate into ions and are thus electrically neutral.

nonvolatile. Does not easily evaporate.

NPO. An abbreviation meaning nothing by mouth (Latin: *nihil per os*).

oliguria. Diminished amount of urination: less than 20 cc/1 hr, 160 cc/8 hrs, 480 cc/24 hrs.

oncotic pressure. Colloid osmotic pressure.

orthopnea. Difficulty in breathing except in an upright position.

osmolality. The concentration of solute per weight or kilogram of solution.

osmolarity. The concentration of solute per volume or liter of solution.

osmosis. The passage of water (solvent) through a semipermeable membrane from an area of lesser concentration to an area of greater concentration of solute; a passive transport system.

osmotic pressure. The pressure developed when two solutions of different concentrations are separated by a semipermeable membrane.

paralytic ileus. Paralysis of the wall of the intestine, involving distention and symptoms of obstruction.

paresthesia. A numbness or a prickling sensation.

parotitis. Inflammation of the salivary glands.

paroxysmal nocturnal dyspnea. A periodically occurring attack of shortness of breath during the night or when in a supine position. Abbr.: PND.

pathophysiological. Related to pathophysiology, the study of an abnormal function.

pCO$_2$. Partial pressure of carbon dioxide (gas).

perfusion. Flow of blood in capillary bed.

pericarditis. Inflammation of the outside layer of the heart.

periphery. Outer part or a surface of a body.

peristalsis. The progressive action caused by the contraction and relaxation of the muscles of the gastrointestinal tract.

pH. A symbol used to express the degree of acidity or alkalinity of the blood; the symbol for hydrogen ion concentration.

phlebothrombosis. Condition of clots in the veins.

plasma. The liquid part of lymph and blood composed of serum and protein substances in solution.

polycythemia. Excess in the number of red corpuscles in the blood.

polydipsia. Excessive thirst.

polyuria. Excessive excretion of urine.

postural blood pressure. Blood pressure as affected by the posture of the body. A decrease of 10 or more points in the systolic pressure from a supine to a standing position can indicate an extracellular fluid deficit.

pO₂. Partial pressure of oxygen.

pressure, osmotic. See osmotic pressure.

proteinate. Principle anion of the extracellular fluid, composed of serum proteins.

RPS. Abbr. for renal pressor substance.

rale. An abnormal sound heard on auscultation of the chest produced by the passage of air through bronchi which contain secretion or exudate or are constricted by spasms.

renin. A protein formed in an ischemic kidney which converts an alpha globulin (hypertensinogen) of the blood into hypertensin (angiotonin), a powerful vasoconstrictor.

rhonchus (pl., rhonchi). A coarse dry rale or rattling in the bronchial tubes.

saline. Combination of sodium, chloride, and water.

saline, normal. A 0.9% salt solution.

semipermeable membrane. A membrane that only permits passage of certain molecules.

sensible loss. Perceptible body fluid and electrolyte loss, such as urine.

sensorium. Degree of mental alertness.

serum. Plasma minus fibrogen, a blood protein.

shock. A state of collapse resulting from acute peripheral circulatory failure. It may occur following hemorrhage, severe trauma, surgery, burns, extracellular fluid deficit, infections, or drug toxicity.

singultus. Hiccoughs.

skin turgor. The degree of tension of the skin.

SMA. Abbr. for sequential multiple analysis; a form of grouping results of several laboratory tests at once. SMA 6 equals six different tests.

SOB. Abbr. for shortness of breath.

sodium. A chemical element that is the major cation of the extracellular fluid.

solute. A substance that is dissolved in a solution.

solution. Liquid containing a dissolved substance.

solvent. The liquid in which another substance (the solute) is dissolved to form a solution.

specific gravity. The weight of a substance compared with an equal part of water. Water is represented by 1.000.

steatorrhea. Fatty stools.

sternal retraction. Strong contraction of the chest muscles in an attempt to pull in more air.

stress mechanism. The body's automatic defenses against stress.

syncope. A transient form of unconsciousness due to cerebral hypoxia; fainting.

tachypnea. Increased frequency of breathing.

tamponade, cardiac. Compression of the heart due to collection of fluid or blood in the pericardium.

TBW. Abbr. for total body water.

third space. An area where extravasated fluid collects and becomes physiologically unavailable to the body.

thromboplastin. A substance found in the tissues or plasma which accelerates clotting of the blood.

tidal volume. The amount of air in one quiet respiration.

tonicity. Measurement of osmotic pressure of a solution.

tortuous. Marked by repeated twists.

toxic. Poisonous or caused by poison.

vasogenic. Related to the vascular system.

VEM. Abbr. for vasoexciter mechanism.

Index

Boldface page numbers indicate tables and figures.